Rima D. Apple

Janet Golden

Editors

The Selling of Contraception

The Dalkon Shield Case, Sexuality, and Women's Autonomy

Nicole J. Grant

Ohio State University Press

Columbus

Library of Congress Cataloging-in-Publication Data

Grant, Nicole J., 1952–
    The selling of contraception : the Dalkon Shield case,
sexuality, and women's autonomy / Nicole J. Grant.
        p.   cm. — (Women and health)
    Includes bibliographical references and index.
    ISBN 0–8142–0572–0
    1. A. H. Robins Company. 2. Dalkon Shield
(Intrauterine contraceptive)—Marketing. 3. Intrauterine
contraceptives—Complications and sequelae.
4. Intrauterine contraceptives industry—United States.
I. Title. II. Series.
HD9995.C64A234   1992
363.9′6′0973—dc20   91–41227
                                                    CIP

Text and jacket design by Kachergis Book Design.
Type set in Garamond No. 3
by Connell-Zeko Type & Graphics, Kansas City, MO.
Printed by Versa Press, East Peoria, IL.

The paper in this book meets the guidelines for permanence
and durability of the Committee on Production Guidelines
for Book Longevity of the Council on Library Resources. ∞

9 8 7 6 5 4 3 2 1

To Bill, Melody, Darren, Courtney, and Casey—with love

All who are morally serious must learn to see, hear, and name the truth of women's lives.

Beverly Wildung Harrison
Our Right to Choose

I do not regard as empty rhetoric a claim that the battles of one group are for all of us.

Stephen J. Gould
The Mismeasure of Man

Contents

Acknowledgments

Research for this study was supported by an American Fellowship from the American Association of University Women. I am grateful to the women of the AAUW for their generosity.

The women who shared their experiences with me for this book have my deepest respect and gratitude. Memories brought forward in their testimonies were accompanied by much sadness and pain. The women told their stories in the hope of helping other women; I have seen that hope realized in the responses of students and other readers of this manuscript who have gained insight and strength from the women's stories.

Bill Grant, my husband and my friend, has given much of himself to make the completion of this work possible. His love, emotional support, and the extra household and child-care burdens he has shouldered on my behalf are deeply appreciated. I am grateful to my son, Darren Hoffman, for the many sacrifices he has made over the years that have contributed substantially to my ability to carry on my work. His understanding, encouragement, and friendship have given me great comfort. My daughter, Courtney Grant, and my son, Casey Grant, have brought great joy to my life in the years it has taken to complete this project. I am grateful to them for all the hugs and kisses that have sweetened my days. I thank them also for the many hours they tried to play quietly so that I could work and be with them, too.

Several people have read versions of this manuscript and have given encouragement and thoughtful critiques. I especially want to thank Sarah Elbert, Jim Geschwender, Bob Bach, Barbara Katz Rothman, David Goode, Holly Blake, Peggy Riley, Debbie Wood, Bob Lilly, Mark Wren, Keith Hedlund, Simon Dinitz, Sybil Shainwald, Charlotte Dihoff, and Nancy Woodington for their respective contributions. While I share responsibility for the strengths of this work with many people, I am solely responsible for its limitations.

These acknowledgments would not be complete without mention of four individuals whose influence in earlier years of my life helped bring me to the point that I could write this book. My grandmother, Gertrude Godfrey, taught me by her courageous example what it meant to be a strong woman and a survivor. She also taught me to read. Her gifts have sustained me through many long and difficult years since her death. Two of my grade school teachers were particularly influential in helping me develop self-esteem and confidence in my abilities to reason and to write: I thank Dorrit Cummings and Estelle Cole of the Glenwood Avenue Elementary School. I am also grateful to my friend Jody Walker for helping me to regain my strength and to create a new life for myself at a time when I felt that too much had been lost. Freedom means so much.

Finally, I want to give special thanks here to three women whose lives have enriched my own beyond measure. For their wisdom, courage, sisterhood, and love, I thank my friends Sarah Elbert, Debbie Wood, and Peggy Riley.

Introduction

This book began as a sociological investigation of the case of the Dalkon Shield. More than four million women worldwide used the Dalkon Shield intrauterine device. Hundreds of thousands of those women were injured by it; many died. The events surrounding the case reflected the complexity of relationships that routinely affect the health and sexuality of women, including particular gender arrangements, particular economic, political, and race relations, and a particular health care delivery system that is global in its reach. I initiated this study to discover precisely how these social and historical conditions influenced the women who used the Dalkon Shield.

Public and professional interest in this case focused primarily on the actions of the manufacturer, the A. H. Robins Corporation. Two important books were published in 1985, each carefully documenting the history of corporate conduct—and misconduct—in the handling of the case. Morton Mintz published *At Any Cost: Corporate Greed, Women, and the Dalkon Shield;* Susan Perry and Jim Dawson published their investigation entitled *Nightmare: Women and the Dalkon Shield.* While those works demonstrated that the actions of the corporation substantially contributed to the risks associated with the use of the Dalkon Shield, they did not explain why women used the Dalkon Shield in the first place, nor why many women continued to use the device—sometimes for many years—after the risks were known.

Women who used the Dalkon Shield have been viewed simplistically as passive victims of professional and corporate conduct. That analysis needs to be reconsidered, with attention given to women as agents in making contraceptive decisions within the larger social and historical contexts informing their lives. Women have, historically, actively practiced procreative control. Within the structural relationships that circumscribe their lives, women exercise some choice and some control over the methods of contraception they will use. The National Women's

Health Network estimated that 60 percent of Dalkon Shield insertions were initiated by patient request. This book gives careful attention to the relationship between the element of choice and the social conditions limiting it.

Implicit in the work thus far produced on this case is the assumption that the risks associated with the Dalkon Shield were incidental to that device alone. I examined the history of other birth control methods to discover risks—both physical and social—in other products available to women today. Other areas that underwent close scrutiny were: ideological considerations that routinely influence contraceptive development and use; material risks identified in the medical literature for the Dalkon Shield and other products; routine professional practices at the level of the corporation, the state, and the health care system; and normative social relationships, both public and private. My purpose was to discover the range of considerations that, in relationship to one another, yielded exposure to risks with the Dalkon Shield, and to evaluate those risks as either incidental to that case or more generalized in their influence on the health and well-being of women.

My methodological approach involved working from the ground up and from the top down to answer two primary questions. First, why did women of diverse backgrounds use the Dalkon Shield? Second, was this case an aberration, or did it reflect normal relationships and routine practices within its sociohistorical context? To answer the first question I conducted a series of seventeen oral history interviews, twelve of them with women who had used the Dalkon Shield. Nine of the twelve had been injured, and three had not. Four of my interviews were with women who used intrauterine devices other than the Dalkon Shield. All four of those women reported that they had suffered some injury or infection, although one woman equivocated, claiming that she had never had a problem with an IUD and yet acknowledging that her IUD had been removed by a physician because he claimed she had an inflammation in her uterus. One of the four, who was severely injured, did not know what type of IUD she had used. She thought she probably had a Copper 7, but she was not certain. She was very young at the time of the interview and had received her IUD many years after the Dalkon Shield was allegedly removed from the market in the United States. Nevertheless, the possibility that her IUD was a Dalkon Shield cannot be absolutely ruled out. The seventeenth interview was with a woman who said that she had never used birth control, although in the course of the interview she said that she had tried rhythm, she had been given birth control pills when she was an unmarried teenager "to regulate her period," her husband had tried condoms during their marriage, and she ultimately had a tubal ligation following her fourth pregnancy.

The sample design for this project followed the pattern suggested by Glaser and Strauss for the generation of grounded theory using theoretical sampling.[1] The initial group of six respondents constituted a convenience sample. The women knew about my interest in women's experiences with the Dalkon Shield, and were willing to talk to me about their own. The sample expanded in a snowball effect, with four respondents contacting me after hearing about the project from women who had already been interviewed. In addition, I placed advertisements in several newspapers announcing that a doctoral candidate wanted to interview women about their experiences with the Dalkon Shield. Two women who answered decided not to participate. Two others lived far away, and travel could not be arranged at a time convenient to them. One woman who volunteered to be interviewed canceled her appointment. Seven women who answered advertisements were included in the seventeen interviewed. All of the women who were not interviewed had used the Dalkon Shield, and all said that they had been injured. Two interviews were lost, one because it was inaudible on tape, and hundreds of miles of travel would have been required to do a second interview with the respondent. The second was eliminated because the respondent knew too much about the project beforehand, and the influence of that prior knowledge was evident in her discussion. The inaudible interview was with a woman who had used the Dalkon Shield but had not been injured; the eliminated interview was with a woman who had used another intrauterine device.

All interviews were shaped by the flow of consciousness of the narrators in response to open-ended questions. Respondents were asked what their lives had been like at the time that they used the method they discussed, and what their experience with that method had been. Any additional questions asked were to facilitate renewed flow of consciousness or clarify points raised by the narrator.

The interviews were transcribed, and all identifying information was edited. The names of the respondents were changed by a method that was completely subjective. Pseudonyms bear no resemblance to the names of the persons interviewed. Quotations were selected from the interviews to illustrate the complexity of considerations identified by these women.

To answer the second primary research question, "Is this case an aberration or does it reflect routine conditions?" I studied the development of contraceptives in general, with particular attention to developments in the late 1950s and 1960s. This involved intensive study of four sources: medical journals, family planning literature, popular magazines, and government investigations of contraceptive products by the Food and Drug Administration, the House of Representatives, and the Senate. Textual analysis of these sources supplemented that of women's oral testimonies, in which this same question was considered with reference to routine conditions in personal life.

The textual analysis of the initial interviews with women made it necessary to consult particular published sources. The history of contraceptives was extremely important to the history of the Dalkon Shield. Many women had experienced problems with oral contraceptives. Many women mentioned reading about problems with the pill in women's magazines, and others said they learned about the Dalkon Shield from those articles. Consequently, I researched the popular magazines of the period 1960–75 to learn what information had been available to women at that time. The magazine articles yielded names of experts who were frequently quoted regarding the safety and efficacy of contraceptive products. I read the major published works by those experts to understand the literature that was available to women who may have read more extensively about contraception at the time. Because much of that published work was written by physicians who dispensed contraceptive information directly to women in their professional practice, the reading of those works yielded some insight into the relationship between women and physicians.

Mention was frequently made in published sources of government activities in regard to contraceptive research, development, and regulation. I read the reports of advisory councils to the U.S. Food and Drug Administration and analyzed the texts of those reports to understand the philosophical and practical motivations that influenced decision making by that agency. I read the transcripts of congressional hearings to discover and analyze the experts' positions as expressed in their testimonies.

The often contradictory testimonies of physicians in the FDA reports, in the congressional hearings, and in published sources led me to examine what had been published directly in medical journals. I consulted the *Index Medicus* from the years 1955 to 1987 and located all the articles pertinent to the Dalkon Shield as well as all the articles on contraception published prior to the Dalkon Shield's arrival on the market. I also read many of the articles published after the Dalkon Shield was no longer marketed in the United States, including those that dealt with the Shield, with other IUDs, and with other methods of contraception. From a textual analysis of that literature I discovered that the safety and efficacy of all contraceptive products were under debate in the medical profession. Proponents on each side of the safety debate—in reference to all forms of contraception discussed—often held steadfastly to their claims that the safety issue had been resolved by scientific studies. Medical researchers' value judgments were apparent in the texts of their debates.

Quotations from interviews, published works, and government documents were selected by two criteria. First, all quotations used to illustrate a dominant point of view were typical of comments frequently appearing in the data. In no case did I extract the most extreme example and offer it as representative of a particular point of view. Second, in the case of exceptional findings, reflecting isolated points of view, each such quotation is identified as exceptional. The full scope of the debates is included in this book. I have attempted to present all conflicts and contradictions as clearly as possible, and at the same time to reflect the confusion the many debates generated.

I designed this project with the intent of generating theory grounded in the data. I knew that the Dalkon Shield case raised many questions about the relationship of women's experiences *as women* to our experiences as women of particular races, classes, and countries. I knew that Dalkon Shields had been dumped in Third World countries after they were withdrawn from the market in the United States, and I suspected that they may have been dumped on poor women within the United States as well. It seemed that the risks must have been intensified by the cumulative effects of race, class, country, and gender. I also knew, however, that many socially privileged women in the United States had used the Dalkon Shield, that many had been injured, and that some had died. I knew that in the United States even the most privileged women complained that medical care was inadequate, claiming that physicians, who were usually male, were arrogant, sexist, and insensitive to women's needs. Nevertheless, I expected that my study would dispel my confusion by yielding a clearer picture of the hierarchy of women's oppression, with the experiences of differently oppressed women being sharply divergent.

For practical reasons I was unable to interview women in any country other than the United States. A representative sample of women who used the Dalkon Shield would have to include women from eighty countries. Because the U.S. government and corporations and family planning organizations based in the United States have extensive influence in those eighty countries, my study of the medical literature, the family planning literature, and government documents may have some relevance to women internationally. My study of the personal lives of women, however, is limited to the specific social and historical context of the United States. Even there, however, it is not intended to be representative of all women who used the Dalkon Shield, nor of all women who used contraceptives at the time that the Dalkon Shield was available. The sample is strictly theoretical. I hope that my analysis will prove useful to a broad population of women.

When I began this project I shared with women of various feminist perspectives a desire to understand the relationships of different women to each other with reference to class, race, country, gender, and sexual oppression. I found that theory was not well formulated on this issue, and I wanted to use this project to contribute to an ongoing process of theoretical inquiry. Therefore I set out with open-ended questions designed to direct me to theoretical premises. I hoped then, and I hope now, that this work will be useful to feminists who share my concern with the generation of theory that explains the similarities and differences among women's experiences and needs as we struggle to bring about global social change on our collective behalf.

In chapter 6 I consider the recent work of feminists of various perspectives as it relates to birth control, sexuality, and the autonomy of women. Among the strengths of feminist scholarship is that it is dynamic and dialectical. I owe a great debt to the many women who have been struggling for decades with the same difficult questions I have attempted to address. It has been a challenge to write the findings of this project as though those findings flowed logically from a start to a finish. The collective work of feminists has influenced the development of the project in many ways at every stage of its development. I include my review of the literature at the end of this manuscript because I returned to that literature after completing my study to reconsider my own theoretical premises in relation to those of my colleagues and mentors. I have done so with deep appreciation for all that I have gained in insight and in courage from the women whose work has preceded my own.

It is an important feminist premise that researchers should disclose the inevitable biases that inform our work. One of my biases is that I firmly believe objectivity to be impossible in scientific endeavors as long as scientists are human. We all bring values to our work, and those values inform the form and content of all that we do. I found little that I would consider objective in any of the data I analyzed for this project. The professional and scientific literature reflected the values, opinions, and subjective judgments of the persons who did the studies and wrote the findings and conclusions. The actions of the state were influenced by the values and subjective opinions of the persons who negotiated policy and the persons who conducted studies. The stories of women were no more or less subjective than the work of professionals, and my own treatment of the project is equally subjective. My values shaped it and influenced my analysis and conclusions. I value health and quality of life for women. I value both fertility and procreative choice. I have made my own risk/benefit assessment of contraceptives and of the social context in which they are developed and used with reference to those values. I have made every effort to be as honest and accurate in my analysis as possible. It is my hope that the values and experiences informing my work have strengthened the validity of the project. My own experiences with the Dalkon Shield—and the pain and suffering of several of my friends who had the device—motivated me to want to know the whole truth about the conditions that contributed to that tragedy. A personal need to know has pushed me to my limits in the search for truth. In the chapters that follow I have presented the truth as I understand it. I hope the reader will find the work useful.

I Birth Control and the Health Care System

Complex historical processes, both technological and social, helped increase power, prestige, and the professional authority of the medical profession in the United States in the early twentieth century. The social position of physicians in the nineteenth century was approximately equal to that of two other groups of healers—women in the home and lay healers. According to Paul Starr, medicine was considered an inferior profession "or at least a career with inferior prospects." Physicians did not, at that time, have the socially recognized authority to "command deference" from their patients or from the larger society.[1]

Urbanization forced many people to rely upon professional services; the development of the telephone and mechanized transportation made the services of professionals more accessible to larger populations; and science began to replace religion as the source of knowledge and hope for the future of humanity. Starr wrote, "People began to regard science as a superior and legitimate way of explaining reality. . . . The less one could believe one's own eyes—and the new world of science continually prompted that feeling—the more receptive one became to seeing the world through the eyes of those who claimed specialized, technical knowledge, validated by communities of their peers."[2]

The discovery of the germ theory of disease and the development of diagnostic technology dramatically increased the dependence of the public on the expertise of the physician. The authority of physicians was increased by what Starr called "mechanisms of legitimation." Medical schools' curricula were standardized, and the licensing of physicians demonstrated that a community of peers validated claims to special expertise. Science offered new hope that the duration and quality of human life could be increased, and physicians became "the emissaries of science."[3]

During the Progressive Era, the authority of physicians extended to control over medications. Starr explained:

> Between 1900 and 1910 three changes enabled the medical profession to wrest control of the flow of pharmaceutical information . . . muckraking journalists joined physicians in a crusade for regulation of patent medicines as part of a general assault on deceptive business practices . . . the AMA finally acquired the financial resources to mount a major effort against patent medicine makers . . . and drug makers were forced to recognize that they depended increasingly on doctors to market their drugs because of the public's increased reliance on professional opinion in decisions about medicine.[4]

The social transformation of American medicine had important consequences for women who wanted to control their procreative power. Traditionally the care of women's health had been shared by a community of women. During childbirth women were attended by female members of their own households or families and by local midwives. Techniques for preventing or spacing births were learned and practiced within the community of women.[5] Methods of birth control over which women had some autonomy included prolonged lactation, homemade cervical barriers, spermicidal douches, chemical, herbal, or mechanical abortifacients, and infanticide. Men had some autonomous control over the use of condoms, withdrawal, and infanticide, but this gave men limited control over women's procreative power. A man who so chose could have prevented his monogamous sexual partner from becoming pregnant. Middle-class men in the nineteenth century may have put considerable pressure on women to have abortions, perhaps at times forcing women not to remain pregnant.[6] But as long as the autonomous prevention or termination of pregnancy by women remained possible, it would have been quite difficult for a man to force a woman to give birth. As the control of health care passed from a community of women to physicians and the state, autonomous control of procreative power by women was increasingly eroded. Women lost control over procreative power as they lost control of health care in general, as providers and as recipients.

State intervention in these matters coincided with the transformation of American medicine and the development of industrial capitalism.

The first laws prohibiting abortion were passed in the midnineteenth century. Changes in official attitudes toward abortion during the nineteenth century are frequently explained by social scientists as a result of demographic changes: a primarily rural, agrarian population was being transformed into a primarily urban, industrial population. Kristin Luker argued, however, that physicians acting out of self-interest played a leading role in the antiabortion campaign of that era. Seeking to increase their authority over health matters, they used the abortion issue as an opportunity to draw attention to their scientific expertise. At the time, the interruption of a pregnancy before quickening was not considered immoral. Even the Catholic church defined abortion as the interruption of pregnancy after quickening. Birth control methods used after conception but before quickening were considered emmenagogues, methods for bringing on a delayed menses, not abortifacients. Physicians in the midnineteenth century claimed that they, through scientific methods, had "discovered" that life began at the moment of conception. They used that argument to support their assertion that any termination of pregnancy was immoral and should be outlawed.[7]

According to James C. Mohr, abortion was practiced by many people of all social classes in the midnineteenth century. Mohr wrote, "Before 1840 abortion was perceived in the United States primarily as a recourse of the desperate. . . . After 1840, however, evidence began to accumulate that the social character of the practice had changed. A high proportion of the women whose abortions contributed to the soaring incidence of that practice in the United States between 1840 and 1880 appeared to be married, native born, Protestant women, frequently of middle- or upper-class status." Demographers claim that the drop in the nation's birthrate after 1840 was brought about by a steep decline in fertility among the privileged classes of native-born whites. According to Mohr, husbands cooperated with their wives, paying for expensive abortions that their wives could not have procured without their help. In some cases, Mohr suggests, the "help" of husbands may have been overzealous, forcing some women to have abortions they did not want. Overall, however, Mohr viewed midnineteenth-century abortion as a companionate effort on the part of couples "to express their sexuality and mutual affections, on the one hand, and to limit their fertility, on the other."[8]

Feminists in the midnineteenth century were alarmed at the apparently rising numbers of abortions. Advocating abstinence instead of abortion or contraception, feminists blamed men for sexually exploiting women through unchecked "sensualism." They viewed abortion as a symptom of women's sexual oppression, not as a means of escaping it. According to Mohr, antiabortion and antifeminist physicians used "the refusal of feminists to advocate abortions" to strengthen their own argument that the practice should be outlawed.[9]

The nineteenth-century antiabortion campaign was ultimately successful. By 1900 abortion could not legally be obtained anywhere in the United States at any stage of pregnancy.[10] The Comstock Law of 1873 banned the interstate mailing of birth control information and contraceptives, further curtailing autonomous use of effective methods of limiting fertility. The passing of licensure laws for the practice of medicine and surgery combined with these factors to push alternatives to compulsory parenthood underground.

With the rapid development of industrial capitalism at the turn of the century, public interest in birth control changed. Professionals and reformers who had opposed the use of birth control in the nineteenth century joined in an effort to make it legal again. As the captains of industry amassed fortunes, the gap between classes was widening. Millions of immigrants joined disfranchised American-born blacks and poor whites in the work force. Urban industrial areas were crowded; provisions for sanitation were negligible. Men, women, and children worked in dangerous and debilitating conditions for long hours at low pay. The middle classes feared the spread of disease and the possibility of revolution.

Progressive reformers turned to science for answers to the social problems of their time. The scientific community attempted to find justifications in nature for the class struggle that had emerged through industrial capitalist development. The social world was viewed as the product of evolutionary change. Science was the source of progress, and industrial capitalist expansion was its manifestation. Individuals who succeeded within that economic milieu were more "fit" to survive; the poor were losing the battle for survival because they were weak and "degenerate." Immigration of hundreds of thousands of indigent people, and the combined concentration of wealth and falling birthrates in the middle and upper classes, caused the poor to outnumber the socially comfortable. The middle classes could not correct this imbalance by having more children themselves without seriously jeopardizing their economic position. Birth control and sterilization for the poor were considered "humane" weapons in the war against "race suicide."[11]

The Comstock Law remained in effect for sixty-five years. Despite the legal and social barriers to contraceptive use, the fertility rate dropped, continuing a trend begun in the early nineteenth century. Public demand for birth control increased during the first four decades of the twentieth century, particularly during the Great Depression. Individuals aggressively sought measures to control their procreative power, and eugenicists and social reformers sought to alleviate social problems through birth control programs. The Comstock Law did not prohibit the *manufacture* of contraceptive products, and manufacturers made substantial profits selling products that were often ineffective and dangerous.[12] Physicians and Progressive reformers joined in opposing the unchecked power of manufacturers, and sought to bring contraceptives, as well as other pharmaceutical products, under physicians' control. These groups turned to the state in their successful effort to mandate those changes.

By the time the Planned Parenthood Federation of America was founded in 1942, just four years after the Comstock Law was repealed, social control had become deeply entrenched as a major objective of the birth control movement, but the language of eugenics had been modified in response to Nazism. Linda Gordon explained:

> PPFA spokespeople declared health the major immediate objective of birth control work. . . . Clearly birth control did contribute to health. The PPFA's emphasis, however, was not on individual welfare but on individuals as items in social planning—"human resource management." During World War II many social scientists contributed analyses of the over-all weaknesses and

strengths of the human resources of the United States and its enemies. . . . Considering human beings as "resources" they viewed people as instrumen talities toward ends defined by rulers, and the PPFA health emphasis shared that orientation.[13]

With the rapid expansion of U.S. imperialism between 1945 and 1960, the consequences of the material interests and ideology informing birth control politics extended to international populations.

According to Heidi Hartmann, demographic changes apparent since the 1950s have altered women's lives considerably. Women have been marrying later, having fewer children, divorcing more frequently, and spending less time living in families and being mothers.[14] Demographers link the fall in fertility which began in the 1960s to delayed marriages, increased labor force participation for married women, and the attainment of higher levels of education for women.[15] According to Hartmann, more women gained some autonomy from the old patriarchal family relationships as a result of those changes. These factors may help to explain why so many women welcomed the birth control "revolution" of the 1960s, seeing in it the promise of deliverance from compulsory motherhood at a time when compulsory motherhood threatened the promise of increasing autonomy for women.[16]

All these historical transformations combined to create the conditions for the birth control "revolution" of the 1960s. But those conditions alone were insufficient to assure the passage of control over procreative power from individuals to professionals and the state. The birth control methods available prior to the 1960s, with the exception of the diaphragm, were available without prescription. While state policy circumscribed individual autonomy to some extent, the transformation from autonomous private control to professional control could not be complete until methods of birth control—and their use— could be brought under direct professional supervision. The discovery of oral contraceptives in the late 1950s was a major step in that direction.

According to Barbara Seaman, health risks with the use of estrogens were documented as early as 1896, when scientists first discovered that estrogen was potentially carcinogenic. Seaman wrote, "By 1938, when Sir Charles Dodds in England synthesized DES—the first inexpensive estrogen product taken by mouth—hundreds of studies on the role of estrogen in carcinogenesis had already been published."[17] Despite the knowledge that estrogens were potentially deadly, oral contraceptives containing high doses of estrogen were heralded as a source of "salvation" for mankind. Dr. John Rock, codeveloper of the "Pill," explained his reason for promoting its development. He wrote:

> Population research is the name given to efforts to know more about all the factors of human reproduction and how best to modify them so that, harmlessly and effectively, conception may, at will, be agreeably precluded as a possible consequence of coitus. Why bother? Because there are already more people on earth than presently utilized resources can properly care for and because Malthus was right when he conservatively remarked, about 175 years ago, that "moral restraint is of dubious effectiveness."[18]

History does not support the assertion that "restraint" has to be imposed on people to effect fertility regulation. Cross-cultural studies by anthropologists reveal that interest in the control of procreative power by individuals is and always has been widespread. The use of abortion and infanticide has been widely documented. Customs of delayed marriage and celibacy have been linked to the effort to limit fertility. Prolonged lactation has been widely used to space pregnancies. The use of condoms dates to antiquity.[19] Improvements in condoms and their mass production after the discovery of the vulcanization of rubber in 1880 may help to explain why fertility rates continued to drop despite the Comstock Law and antiabortion legislation.

Norman Himes wrote in 1936 that conception control was "older than propaganda movements." In the introduction to *Medical History of Contraception,* he referred to the "universal aim of controlled *paternity* [emphasis mine]," although he acknowledged that "the chief 'preventive' or birth-limiting check in primitive society was abortion." Himes cited several methods in which male participation was customary, including "delayed marriage and celibacy . . . sex tabus limiting the time and frequency of connection, pre-puberty coition . . . [and] sex perversion."

He also described subincision, a technique whereby an opening was surgically introduced at the base of the penis, causing semen to be emitted from the base, not the end of the penis.[20]

Himes described a number of methods used by women to prevent conception. He claimed that black women in Guyana and Martinique used lemon juice as a spermicide and cut lemons in half and hollowed them out for use as cervical caps. In the Middle East, he claimed, women used pomegranates for the same purpose. He also described an intravaginal condom used by Guyanese women and made from "okra-like pods held in the vagina, closed end toward the cervix, open end at the vaginal opening." Himes cited the use of leaves and herbs taken orally, but claimed they were "undoubtedly ineffective . . . since no drug taken by mouth is known to western science that will prevent conception or abort." Himes did not consider that women may have known about and used effective methods about which medical scientists were ignorant. He was writing, after all, before the discovery by western scientists of oral contraceptive compounds derived from plants, and before feminist historians began to discover and publish the history of women as healers and the history of women's lives and women's support networks. In addition, his title makes his intent to publish a *medical*—not a *social*—history of contraception clear.[21]

Aware, nevertheless, of women's historic motivation to control procreative power, Himes wrote, "Women of all times have longed to control their maternal, biological function; they have wanted both fertility and sterility, each in its appointed time and place. This fear of slavery to pregnancy has been to many women like a ghost stalking the corridor of time, always present, yet always elusive; sometimes placated, but more often threatening. Often, pathetically, women have hit upon the ineffective and injurious; and only lately has science consciously begun to help them." To underscore his point, he cited an entry in a Chinese medical text that he estimated first appeared between 1506 and 1521. The author wrote, "As a rule, in contraceptive prescriptions, many use dangerous and violent ones, so that we constantly have cases that do not recover.

Really then the injury from childbirth is not as great as the injury from preventing childbirth."[22]

Recently anthropologists have discovered many indigenous fertility regulation methods (IFRMs). Most of those methods are controlled by women and communicated intergenerationally and through midwives or other female healers and herbalists. Lucile Newman identified a set of context variables deriving from social and cultural relationships that affect fertility. She wrote:

> In some societies, inheritance of land and economic continuity are central determinants of reproduction. . . . For others, the key issues are "purity" of lineage and ritual continuity. . . . for still others, the quality of life of each child and each child's opportunities dominate. . . . the anthropological perspective . . . addresses what issues influence kinship and union formation, what kinds of social control and individual regulation are acceptable to people, and what initiatives are acceptable for personal regulation of fertility.[23]

In short, anthropologists have learned that individuals do what they can with what they have to affect fertility when they perceive it to be in their interests to do so. Fertility regulation methods are often used in defiance of laws, customs, and religious mandates. Belief systems are sometimes creatively modified to accommodate the use of fertility regulation.[24] Indigenous fertility regulation involves methods for enhancing fertility as well as those intended to limit it.[25]

In desperate situations, where alternatives are limited, women often resort to violent and potentially lethal methods of birth control.[26] There is evidence, however, to suggest that many of the indigenous methods of birth control used by communities of women are both effective and relatively noninjurious, including some methods of abortion. Many Third World women today continue to use indigenous methods passed on through female support networks, especially those transmitted by their own mothers and grandmothers. Suspicious of foreign products and the motives of persons disseminating them, many women refuse to risk injury for the sake of the reputed enhanced effectiveness of commercial methods. Anthropologists have found that many indigenous methods have properties now recognized by western medicine as effective in preventing pregnancy, a finding that challenges the claim by western scientists and social scientists that indigenous methods are based on superstition or magic.[27]

Within western industrialized countries during the last hundred years, women have risked injury, arrest, and death to exercise procreative control when state policy and social transformations made the practice of birth control a potentially lethal endeavor. In the United States, immigration, migration, and urbanization contributed to women's isolation from traditional female support networks. Ideological support for medical science as progressive and the concurrent rejection of nonmedical science as unscientific further alienated women from the knowledge of their foremothers.

In the first seven decades of the twentieth century, women in the United States had to rely increasingly on illegal abortion services performed by strangers and on contraception supplied by industry and professionals when private attempts to prevent conception failed, or when partners would not or could not help to prevent conception effectively. Self-help strategies controlled by women or by women and their sexual partners gradually gave way to birth control efforts that depended on the purchase of commodities that were often expensive. The state became the locus of birth control negotiations, and many men and women were unrepresented there.

According to Linda Gordon, many more women died from illegal abortions than from legal abortions.[28] The Boston Women's Health Collective offered an explanation: "Abortionists emphasized speed and their own protection. They often didn't use anesthesia because it took too long for women to recover, and they wanted women out of the office as quickly as possible. Some abortionists were rough and sadistic. Almost no one explained what was happening, discussed birth control techniques or took adequate precautions against hemorrhage or infection."[29] Despite these conditions, many millions of women risked their lives and their reputations to obtain abortions. According to the Boston Women's Health Collective, "In the 1950's about a million illegal abortions a year were performed in the U.S., and over a thousand women died each year as a result. Women came into emergency wards only to die of widespread abdominal infections, victims of botched or unsanitary abortions. Many women who recovered from such infection found themselves sterile and painfully ill."[30]

In the 1960s professionals writing on birth control did not present the image of women so desperate to prevent conception that they would risk their lives. Their image of women was one of laziness, stupidity, and reluctance to use birth control when it was available to them. In 1925 physicians had sought to secure control over the dissemination of contraceptives in order to *limit* the conditions under which they could be used.[31] By 1960 they were seeking to control the dissemination and the use of birth control to *broaden* conditions for effective use.

The failure of birth control methods in the 1960s was consistently blamed on women. In 1965, four years before Barbara Seaman published *The Doctors' Case against the Pill,* she wrote an article in the *Ladies' Home Journal* entitled "Tell Me Doctor: 'Why Did Birth Control Fail Me?'" Seaman wrote, "Scientifically speaking, the problem of conception control has been solved. Pills and intrauterine coils work almost perfectly. Diaphragms are almost as reliable. And, for women whose monthly cycles are regular, the rhythm method is more dependable than is popularly believed. But, as Christopher Tietze, Director of the National Committee on Maternal Health, says, 'The main reason for contraceptive failure is failure to use the contraceptive!'"[32]

In 1969 Laurence Lader published "Why Birth Control Fails" in *McCall's.* He wrote, "Many women are still frighteningly irresponsible about birth control and are ignorant or lazy enough to use methods like rhythm and withdrawal, which hardly deserve to be ranked as contraception."[33] Lader's charge that the use of the highly complicated rhythm method is an indication of laziness might be inappropriate, but the charge that women were responsible for birth control failure was typical. Garrett Hardin, whose book, *Birth Control,* appeared the next year, wrote, "The dream of 'every child a wanted child' . . . is a dream that is already within our grasp. . . . We have everything we need now. Technologically, perfect birth control is a reality now. All we have to do is decide to use it."[34]

How "perfect" the new birth control technologies really were was a subject of controversy during the 1960s. Between 1966 and 1969 the U.S. Food and Drug Administration appointed three advisory committees to study two methods of contraception. A report on oral contraceptives was published in 1966, a report on intrauterine devices in 1968, and a second report on oral contraceptives in 1969. In 1970 Senate hearings chaired by Senator Gaylord Nelson convened to discuss whether women were being adequately informed about hazards associated with the pill.

In the introduction to the FDA's 1966 report, the advisory committee noted that oral contraceptives were the first drugs taken "voluntarily over a protracted period for an objective other than for control of disease." Several deaths had been reported in association with oral contraceptives, which were then new drugs that had been marketed in the United States for six years and in Puerto Rico for nine. The advisory committee had been appointed to study the incidence of complications and to consider the adequacy of methods of surveillance and reporting of adverse effects. The philosophy reflected in the report was illustrated by the following quotation from the opening paragraph:

> Probably no substance, even common table salt, and certainly no effective drug can be taken over a long period of time without some risk, albeit minimal. There will always be a sensitive individual who may react adversely to any drug, and the oral contraceptives cannot be made free of such adverse potentials, which must be recognized and kept under continual surveillance. The potential dangers must also be carefully balanced against the health and social benefits that effective contraceptives provide for the individual woman and society.[35]

The committee reported that the principal problem associated with the study of oral contraceptives was that "major deficiencies" existed in the system of surveillance. Physicians did not consistently report adverse effects they saw in patients using the drugs; some incidents were more likely than others to be reported due to "fashions in medical interest rather than the magnitude of a possible hazard"; no one knew how many women actually used the drugs, so neither prevalence nor incidence of adverse effects could be accurately established; there was an alleged absence of control populations of nonusers for comparison; and the researchers were not able to determine the "potential long-term effects which might first appear after discontinuation of the oral contraceptives or even in the progeny of users."[36]

Four task forces were assigned to study efficacy and three areas of potential hazard—thromboembolic disease, carcinogenic potential, and endocrine and metabolic effects. The findings of each task force were published as appendixes to the main body of the committee report; the body of the report included summaries of task force findings and the final recommendations and conclusions of the committee.

The task force on thromboembolic disease found a *lower* than expected incidence of death from that disease reported in women using oral contraceptives than in the general population of women of the same age group. The task force considered two explanations for this: "(1) The oral contraceptives are protective against thromboembolic disease; (2) there has been gross underreporting." The task force hypothesized that underreporting was the more plausible explanation and noted that "physicians are becoming increasingly fearful of reporting deaths or adverse drug reactions because of potential legal reprisal."[37]

The task force on carcinogenic potential claimed that definitive conclusions could not be reached because oral contraceptives had been used for less than ten years. According to their report, "All known human carcinogens require a latent period of approximately a decade." The task force reported that various cancers had been produced in laboratory animals given high dosages of estrogens, but investigators were skeptical about the usefulness of animal studies in predicting human reactions to the same compounds.[38]

The task force on endocrine and metabolic effects found evidence of a possible link between oral contraceptive use and impairment of pituitary-ovarian, pituitary-adrenal, and liver functioning, as well as changes in carbohydrate metabolism. They found that lactation was suppressed when nursing mothers were given estrogens. There were reports of masculinization in some women and in the female fetuses of others who had used oral contraceptives during the early stages of pregnancy. Fetal abnormalities had been found in laboratory animals, but the task force had no data on possible genetic effects in humans.[39]

The advisory committee also identified a potential relationship between oral contraceptive use and ophthalmologic complications, migraine, and "psychological and emotional factors." Again it was claimed that precise data were unavailable.[40]

The task force report on efficacy considered several uses of oral contraceptives, including control of fertility and treatment of amenorrhea, dysmenorrhea, endometriosis, functional uterine bleeding, habitual abortion, and several miscellaneous uses including the treatment of menopausal syndrome, acne, chronic vulvar infections, and psychiatric disorders. The authors expressed ambivalence about the usefulness of the drugs for any end other than fertility control. For that purpose, the report noted, "The efficacy of the combined agents is exceptionally high," and the newer sequential pills were "also highly effective, although to a slightly lesser degree."[41]

Each task force emphasized the need for more and better studies and for improved methods of study and surveillance. The final recommendations of the committee reflected that concern. Of the ten recommendations presented, seven called for direct support of additional studies. The committee sought the implementation of new types of studies, financial support for those studies, and improved methods of communication between government, corporations, and practitioners in order to facilitate more accurate studies. The remaining three recommendations called for changes that would less directly but significantly support the continuing study of the effects of oral contraceptives on human populations. One indicated a need for uniform labeling of all contraceptive drugs; another suggested that the two-year time limit on the prescription of oral contraceptives to individual women be lifted, allowing for indefinite periods of use; and the third called for "simplification of administrative procedures to allow reduction in dosage of already approved compounds."[42] That change would allow researchers to test the effects of lower dosages without waiting for FDA approval.

The committee's concern for limiting administrative procedures was explained in the second paragraph of the introduction to the report. The authors wrote, "The research essential to the development and testing of these compounds is carried out by the drug industry working in close cooperation with the medical profession. It would be indeed unfortunate were such research and testing to be stifled by unnecessarily harsh and inelastic administrative procedures."[43]

The release of that report by the FDA helped make wider and longer use of oral contraceptives by women possible. Between 1965 and 1969 use of the pill doubled.[44] Reports of complications increased dramatically in the popular press as well as in the medical literature.

In 1968 the U.S. Food and Drug Administration appointed a committee to study intrauterine devices. The introduction to the committee's report began:

> Rebirth of interest in the intrauterine devices (IUDs) as an effective, acceptable method of contraception stems from two factors. First is the availability of inert plastics that may be straightened to allow easy insertion and that return to their original shape, in which they are retained within the uterus. Second is the suggestion that the underprivileged woman is more effectively served when the need for recurrent motivation, required in most other forms of contraception, is removed. Several additional advantages of the intrauterine devices commend their use. Although their mode of action in women has not been fully elucidated, the antifertility action cannot be associated with any known systemic effect. Problems of initial distribution and followup are smaller than those associated with the oral contraceptives, and the expense of the intrauterine device is negligible. Whereas intrauterine contraception is not quite as effective as the best oral compounds, its use-effectiveness ratio is more favorable than that of traditional methods of contraception.[45]

That introduction reflected the historical context within which decisions would be made regarding technological methods of contraception in several ways. First, "the suggestion that the underprivileged woman is more effectively served" with a method that requires little motivation on her part reflects professional ignorance of the historical struggle of women to attain the means to control procreative power. It also reflects a class bias, by identifying the "underprivileged" woman as particularly unmotivated. (Class bias is discussed in more detail in chapter 5.) Furthermore, the introduction reflects growing concern about the systemic effects of oral contraceptives, and the concern that women who might decide that the pill was too risky could simply stop taking the drug. The reference to "use-effectiveness" supports both the idea that women are irresponsible when it comes to using contraception effectively, and the concern that both traditional methods of contraception and oral contraceptives leave control of the method in the hands of the woman. *Use-effectiveness* in this report referred to the expected effectiveness of a given method in actual use; the term *technical effectiveness* was used to refer to the expected effectiveness of a given method under carefully controlled laboratory conditions. Professionals sought methods of birth control with the highest possible use-effectiveness. Such methods would necessarily, according to the experts, entail the least possible motivation—and the least possible control—on the part of the woman.

In "Historical Styles of Contraceptive Advocacy," Joyce Berkman wrote, "Reproductive self-determination could be compatible with a woman freely choosing a family of ten children. This was far from the minds of contraceptive proponents, who defined birth control strictly as family limitation."[46] Beverly Wildung Harrison, in her ethical consideration of abortion, used the terms *procreative control* and *procreative choice* for the efforts of women to exercise control over their power to procreate.[47] *Birth control* is the effort to control birth *rates; population control* refers to the control of particular populations. Birth control and population control were the focus of professional efforts by the 1960s; procreative choice for individual women was not on the agenda for a majority of those professionals.

The distinction between procreative choice and population control was illustrated by the 1968 report on intrauterine devices, by the 1969 report on oral contraceptives, and by the 1970 Senate hearings on the pill. The committee studying intrauterine devices was divided into five task forces. One was responsible for studying the biologic action of

IUDs—how they work to prevent pregnancy; another was to study utilization and effectiveness; a third was responsible for studying "inflammatory reactions and warnings"; a fourth studied carcinogenic potential; and the fifth task force studied existing legislation to determine whether it was adequate to govern the handling of IUDs.

The task force on biologic action reported that it had studied rats, rabbits, sheep, swine, cattle, rhesus monkeys, and women. They considered several explanations for IUDs' ability to prevent pregnancy, including damage to or blockage of sperm by the device, increased speed of transport of the ova through the oviducts, overall systemic effects on the body, and localized effects on the uterine lining (endometrium). They found some variation among species, but in *every species* the committee found evidence of inflammation and signs of infection in the endometrium. The task force concluded, "In women there is histological evidence of endometrial inflammation and alterations in the normal endometrial progression during the menstrual cycle; these changes may be sufficient to explain the prevention by IUDs of uterine pregnancies."[48] Inflammation and infection, according to that report, were not merely potential hazards of IUD use—they were quite possibly the necessary effects of IUDs in order for conception to be prevented.

The task force on utilization and effectiveness compared the technical effectiveness and the use-effectiveness of IUDs. According to that report, in other contraceptives the difference between the two rates of effectiveness was the result of "human frailty." The task force found that the use-effectiveness of the IUD approached its technical effectiveness. As stated in the introduction of the advisory committee's report, "recurrent motivation" was unnecessary with an IUD. Unless an IUD was involuntarily expelled, it would remain effective at the technical rate of effectiveness until it was removed by a health care professional. The task force noted that "an IUD will continue to prevent conception if the wearer forgets its presence or if she mistakenly believes that the device has been expelled or removed." The task force did not explain under what conditions a woman might "mistakenly believe" that an IUD had been removed. The idea that control by professionals over the reproductive functions and choices of women was a goal of contraceptive development was, however, implicit.[49]

The task force report on inflammatory reactions deepened the suspicion that infection might be endemic to IUD use. The task force studied autopsy reports and concluded that the deaths of at least four women had probably resulted from IUD-related infections. The report stated the following warnings: (1) "The transcervical insertion of an IUD probably cannot be done without introducing bacteria and in many cases creating an intrauterine infection"; (2) "The incidence of infection is significantly higher within the first month after insertion of a device than in subsequent months"; (3) "The incidence of pelvic infection is higher in women wearing intrauterine devices than in a control population without the devices"; (4) "The rate of pelvic inflammatory disease varied from less than 1 percent in groups of private patients to 8 percent in an indigent clinic group"; (5) "There is an unfortunate tendency for many physicians to discount the need for any but the barest minimum of sterile precautions."[50]

The task force recommended that sterile precautions should be taken in the packaging and handling of intrauterine devices. Although the report expressed dismay that corporations and physicians often chose to ignore recommendations for voluntary compliance with safety precautions, it did not recommend that special legislation be enacted to govern the handling of IUDs.

The task force appointed to study carcinogenic potential found that it had too little data on which to base any definitive conclusions. It recommended that IUD users have semiannual pelvic exams and Pap smears, and that biopsies be performed "where indicated."[51]

The task force on legislation, after reviewing both proposed legislation for prosthetic devices and the findings of the other four task forces, recommended that intrauterine devices should be included in the general legislation that would require manufacturers to apply for preclearance of products and to supply the FDA with data "adequate to support a conclusion that they are safe, effective, and reliable for the usage intended," and reported that it was "opposed to any legislation directed specifically at contraceptive devices."[52] In the opinion of the task force, IUDs would be adequately covered by legislation already governing hearing aids, dental plates, orthopedic shoes, and the like. The recommendations also indicated that, in the task force's opinion, the FDA could depend on the manufacturer's data about the safety of products submitted for preclearance.

The logical discrepancies between the alarming contents of the task force reports, particularly on biologic action and inflammatory reactions, and the conclusions of the report that no special legislation was needed to govern the handling of IUDs, cannot be explained with reference to science or to objectivity. Objectively, IUDs were dangerous. The suspicion that they might work by causing infection could have caused an objective observer to conclude that those devices could not safely be worn by women. As Carol Korenbrat wrote, however, "Although 'risk' can be restricted to the likelihood of the occurrence of an adverse effect, 'safety' is the judgment of the acceptability of risks. . . . The acceptability of risks is a function of the desirability of benefits, and that is a matter of judgment and not of scientific expertise. To make such a decision involves the application of values to facts."[53]

In the FDA's 1969 report on oral contraceptives, the weighing of benefits against risks was explicitly identified as the appropriate process for determining the safety of contraceptive products. In his opening summary Louis Hellman wrote, "Concern about the immediate and long-range side effects of the hormonal contraceptives has increased as scientific investigations have uncovered a host of diverse biologic effects, and as the drugs have become available to increasingly large segments of the population. . . . Adverse reactions are continually reported in the scientific literature and the lay press." Hellman noted the points of contention among professionals about the reports of adverse effects: "Controversy has centered about two areas: the scientific data required to establish an etiologic relation and the balance between acceptable risk and potential benefit." Because reporting of adverse effects by physicians was "fragmentary at best," "it is difficult to separate fact from fiction at the forefront of scientific discovery."[54]

According to the committee's report, the risk to individual users of oral contraceptives was intensified by the considerable time lag between discovery of a problem and the establishment by the scientific community of a causal relationship. In the case of thromboembolic disease, "Eight years were required from the time of the first reported death to establish the relative risk and an etiologic relation to the hormonal contraceptives." Before evaluating the progress made in carrying out the 1966 committee recommendations and issuing new ones, Hellman made the following observation: "The task of balancing the risk against the benefit to the individual and to society must eventually be met. As contraceptive practices spread to all segments of our society, it becomes virtually essential that the requirements of effectiveness and safety, and the desirability of inexpensiveness and lack of association with coitus be satisfied."[55]

The agenda reflected by Hellman's summary led to a conclusion that was logically inconsistent with the findings of the task forces assigned to study adverse effects. Those task forces identified more than seventy adverse reactions that had been associated with the use of oral contraceptives. Those reactions were: delayed menses; amenorrhea; spotting; headache; nausea; gastric distress; vomiting; pelvic cramps; feelings of abdominal fullness; nervousness; anxiety; depression; dizziness; leg cramps; breast tenderness; breast enlargement; unusual fatigue; backache; hirsutism; acne; urticaria; chloasma; weight gain; weight loss; changes in libido; fetal abnormalities; hypersecretion and hyperplasia of the cervical glands; stromal edema; increased vascularity; gross cervical lesions; edema, softening, erosion, or eversion of the cervix; fibrii thrombi; atypical endocervical hyperplasia; severe thinning or regression of the endometrium; changes in enzymatic activity of endometrial tissue; myometrial hypertrophy; dilation of sinusoids and edema in the endometrium; focal areas of cortical stromal fibrosis; thrombi in ovarian and uterine veins; moderate changes in liver function tests in asymptomatic women; jaundice; decreased metabolism of cortisone; interference with the metabolism or detoxification of certain drugs; modification of carbohydrate metabolism with a decrease in glucose tolerance; changes in thyroid function; alterations in adrenocortical function; increase in blood pressure; changes in the chemical composition of blood; alterations in lipid and lipoprotein composition; changes in salt and water metabolism; alteration in zinc, copper, magnesium, and iron metabolism; ureteral dilation after cessation of medication; increased alveolar venliation; decreases in arterial pCO_2; increase in bronchial resistance; increase in histamine; inhibition of gas transfer; progressive pulmonary lesions characterized by an accumulation of macrophages in capillaries, migration of macrophages to the alveolar interstitium and diffuse interstitial pneumonitis; nervous system excitability; interference with thermoregulation; migraine; premature epiphyseal closure; melasma; increased sensitivity to sunlight; male-type partial alopecia; acute colonic lesions; chromosomal abnormalities; increased incidence of seizure in epileptics; abnormal patency of the Eustachian tube; hypertrophic gingivitis; myalgia; collagen disorders; exacerbation of lupus erythematosus; masculinization of female fetuses; infertility of female offspring in rats; and stillbirths in monkeys.

After compiling this dramatic list the committee made eight recommendations. Four sought to strengthen communications and surveillance; two called for more studies; one suggested a national fertility study; and one called for "substantial support [to] be supplied to develop new methods of contraception."[56]

The conclusion of the 1969 report primarily concerned the question of a risk/benefit ratio. The committee defined safety, in fact, with reference to a risk/benefit assessment. The entire conclusion was published as follows:

> Although the Kefauver-Harris Amendment of 1962 indicates that the term "safe" has reference to the health of man, nowhere do they define safety. Discussing this subject before the Subcommittee of the Committee on Government Operations of the House of Representatives, the Commissioner of the FDA pointed out that no effective drug can be absolutely safe. Therefore, evaluating safety of a drug requires weighing benefit against risk.
>
> The Advisory Committee on Obstetrics and Gynecology has continued to assess the risk of oral contraceptives in this light, weighing knowledge of potential hazards against benefit. It has periodically reviewed the labeling of

these compounds, repeatedly advocated strict surveillance by physicians, and recommended the accumulation of additional information about biological action and clinical effects. This report states the benefit of these compounds compared with those of other contraceptives.

Specific risks as well as requisite practices for followup of patients have been detailed in the labeling of all hormonal contraceptives. When these potential hazards and the value of the drugs are balanced, the Committee finds the ratio of benefit to risk sufficiently high to justify the designation safe within the intent of the legislation.[57]

In December 1969, a press release announced hearings "to explore the question whether users of birth control pills are being adequately informed concerning the pill's known health risks." The release said that 8.5 million women were then using oral contraceptives in the United States, and ten million women were using them in other countries. These figures did not include all women who had ever used the pill.[58]

In his opening statement Senator Gaylord Nelson said:

Misinformation has been widely disseminated. For example in the January 1970 issue of *Redbook* magazine we find the following statement: "Because of reports of complications associated with its use, there is much controversy about the safety of the pill. But it is difficult to determine whether there is direct cause and effect relationship, because reports of complications are rare in comparison to the large number of women using the oral contraceptives." An article in *Bride* magazine of December 1969 which will no doubt be read by many young women makes the following claims: "The pill is virtually 100 percent effective. A pill user who has headaches, fatigue or leg cramps often blames these on the pill rather than on overwork or a bad day at home. The pill prevents ovulation with the same hormones that the body produces during pregnancy. The pill is probably the most thoroughly tested drug ever approved for use in this country. Statistically a woman's chance of death during pregnancy is eight times greater than the chance of death from clotting disease."[59]

Nelson's concern that women were insufficiently informed about the risks of using oral contraceptives were countered by Senator Dole, who was concerned that women were being needlessly frightened away from using them. Dole said:

We must not frighten millions of women into disregarding the considered judgement of their physicians. . . . Let us show some sympathy for the beleaguered physicians who must weigh not only the safety and efficacy of alternative methods for a particular woman, but the emotional reactions of that woman which have been generated by sensational publicity and rumored medical advice. . . . It would be unfortunate if efforts to assist American women only served to confuse them. They have already been subjected to heavy doses of alarm and reassurances by the proponents and opponents of the pill in the mass media. Let us hope our investigation can provide some clarity.[60]

Dole's concern was not limited to the need to dispel confusion, however. He added, "I can safely say that I share with the chairman a deep concern for national and world problems of overpopulation and environmental health. It is apparent that at the present time the oral contraceptives are important weapons in the struggle to achieve some control over our ability to multiply ourselves into chaos."[61]

Men on both sides of the debate cited the welfare of women as their focus of concern, but men on both sides of the debate had additional concerns. Dr. Hugh J. Davis, who had a vested interest in promoting intrauterine devices in place of oral contraceptives, made passionate declarations of his concern for women in his testimony against the pill.

No one, as the FDA was careful to point out, has the slightest idea what long-range effects may result from such chronic use of the pill for 15, 20, or even 30 years. It can be said, however, that 9 million women is a very large scale experiment. . . . Is the consumer—the woman—aware of, or even capable of fully understanding all of these complex questions which have puzzled and concerned some of the best brains in medicine for the past decade? . . . I think certainly little attempt has been made either to inform her or to protect her. In many clinics the pill has been served up as if it were no more hazardous than chewing gum.[62]

Yet Dr. Davis' concern did not extend equally to all women. He said:

It is especially tragic that for the individual who needs birth control the most—the poor, the disadvantaged, and the ghetto-dwelling black—the oral contraceptives carry a particularly high hazard of pregnancy, as compared with methods requiring less motivation. . . . it is the suburban middle-class woman who has become the chronic user of the oral contraceptives in the United States in the past decade, getting her prescription renewed month after month and year after year without missing a single tablet. Therein, in my opinion, lies the real hazard of the presently available oral contraceptives.[63]

Davis' testimony illustrated several trends within the health care system that influenced decision making about contraceptives. His attitude toward all women was patronizing; women could not be expected to grapple successfully with the "complex questions" that had concerned "some of the best brains" (presumably the brains of men) "in medicine for the past decade." His class bias, racism, and nationalism were typical of views commonly expressed by professionals interested in birth and population control. But in separating the specifics of women's contraceptive needs by race and class, he conveniently identified a particular need shared by all women—the need for an effective alternative to the pill. Poor women and black "ghetto-dwelling" women needed a method that was more use-effective, he postulated, because they lacked the motivation to take oral contraceptives. Middle-class women needed a different method because they were so intensely motivated that they would take the potent drugs constantly for prolonged periods of time.

Proponents of the alleged safety of oral contraceptives were equally condescending to women. One physician, Robert Kistner, went so far as to testify that the suggestion that a blood clot might occur could cause a woman to develop a clot. He was questioned closely about this.

Q. Doctor, in all your experience, have you ever heard of one case where suggestion induced the formation of a blood clot? Have you ever heard of one case?

A. As diagnosed by what method?

Q. Well, Doctor, does suggestion cause blood clotting? It doesn't, does it doctor?

A. Well, it might. . . . It might. There's a possibility through various adrenal factors and by the excitation of some of the blood clotting mechanisms that it might.

Q. All right. In other words, you can suggest to somebody if they take this they might get a blood clot and the very suggestion would cause a blood clot?

A. It very frequently causes the symptoms which are exactly the same as blood clotting, and that's the reason I asked about the method of diagnosis, because if it were not precise, the incidence would be higher.

Q. Now Doctor, I'm not talking about symptoms; I'm talking about the existence of a clot. Can you suggest the formation of a clot and have it occur in a human being?

A. It might be possible to do so, yes.

Q. Have you ever seen a documented case where somebody made a suggestion that "You are going to get a blood clot," and then it developed?

A. No, I have not.

Q. There's not such a case in all the medical literature, is there?

A. But you asked me if it were possible.

Q. But there has never been a case like that?

A. I know of no such cases.[64]

The testimony of some experts was more credible. Dr. David B. Clark was concerned that obstetrician-gynecologists were not seeing all the stroke victims whose condition might be linked to their use of oral contraceptives. He explained:

> It is not surprising that the question of a relationship between the taking of oral contraceptives and strokes should have been suggested at first largely by neurologists, who would naturally tend to see a greater concentration of these problems than the general physician or obstetrician. The first suggestive case report appeared in 1962, published by Lorentz. In the ensuing 8 years, rather better than 100 have been reported in the world medical literature in varying detail. One gets the impression that there are probably a great many more cases, but this is only an impression. There was, as I have indicated, and there still is, no reliable and continuing system of reporting.[65]

Clark was not concerned that women might develop symptoms by suggestion; he was concerned that physicians might fail to recognize the early warning symptoms of impending pill-related stroke. He said:

> There are some suggestions that the strokes which have occurred in women taking the pill may be different in their manifestations and their method of development from more commonly occurring strokes. . . . In a very few autopsied cases, and very few autopsies are reported, there is microscopic evidence that a slow process of occlusion of arteries and then healing may have been going on in several parts of the brain for some time before a major artery is involved. These changes, in at least a few of the autopsied cases, do not strictly resemble the sort of change one is accustomed to seeing in the commonly occurring strokes with which we are familiar.[66]

He advised that "any woman taking the drugs who begins to have migrainous headaches, in whom previously present migraine is worsened or who experiences disturbances of speech, vision, motor coordination, or sensation, should stop the drugs at once."[67]

Dr. Roy Hertz was critical of the "world-wide enthusiasm for the pill."

The widely recognized urgency of the population problem served to supplement existing industrial pressures for the hasty exploitation of these remarkable new agents. These influences led to a most prompt and indulgent endorsement of the pill not only by our regulatory agencies but also by notably responsible groups dedicated to the advancement of birth control. There was thus created a world-wide enthusiasm for the pill which to this day has hampered a truly comprehensive and objective evaluation of its merits and demerits.[68]

In Hertz's risk/benefit analysis, risks weighed most heavily. He said, "In view of the general availability of somewhat less effective but even more feasible alternative methods of contraception, readily supplemented by the surgical interruption of unaverted pregnancies by qualified physicians, I can visualize only a rare circumstance indeed in which I would recommend estrogen-progestogen mixtures for contraceptive use."[69]

In his closing comments, Senator Dole expressed dismay at the state of alarm the hearings had caused.

Headlines such as "Pill Takers Held More Cancer Prone" were the hallmarks of January's hearings. Testimony raising questions casting doubt dominated the hearings and headlines. Risks predominated over benefits. Fears were emphasized over effectiveness. These hearings have amplified the doubts and uncertainties the American woman has had about oral contraceptives. Another unfortunate aspect of these hearings is that no new knowledge has been disclosed.[70]

Senator Nelson had a different opinion: "Although very little of the information presented here or perhaps none of it was new to experts in the field, quite obviously a lot of it was not known to the practicing physician who prescribes the pill and the public who consumes it."[71]

The debate continued after the hearings were over. As *Time* magazine reported, "The most recent assessments of the Pill were given last month to the American Association of Planned Parenthood Physicians and the American College of Physicians. No two assembled experts agreed completely on the relative advantages and risks of the Pill, or in defining the patients for whom they would prescribe or proscribe it."[72]

In 1969 and 1970 men on each side of the debate published books in which they considered the pill's safety. Morton Mintz, a journalist for the *Washington Post,* published *The Pill: An Alarming Report,* warning consumers of the dangers that had been associated with the drugs. He traced information on the pill from the time that it was first introduced, showing that experts had equivocated about its safety, and explained the FDA's use of a risk/benefit assessment to arrive at conclusions inconsistent with the facts uncovered in their study.[73]

Paul Vaughan wrote a book critical of the pill in which he said, "The sheer diversity of effects reported to be possibly linked with the pill would be enough to scare most women off and send them back thankfully to coitus interruptus, the cap or the condom." He noted that ignorance within the medical profession compounded the problem, making an accurate assessment of the actual risks impossible: "Explanations for the side-effects which are reported in such bewildering variety constantly founder on one basic difficulty: in the present state of medical knowledge it is impossible to be sure exactly what is happening to the steroids in the pill once they get into the body. This is not only because not enough is known about the pill. Not enough is known about the body either."[74]

Physicians who were proponents of the safety of the pill used the authority of their professional credentials as weapons in the battle with the pill's opponents. In 1969 Dr. Alan F. Guttmacher published *Birth Control and Love: The Complete Guide to Contraception and Fertility.* Opposite the title page was a listing of Dr. Guttmacher's credentials—"President, Planned Parenthood Federation of America; Former Director of Obstetrics and Gynecology at Mount Sinai Hospital, New York; Emeritus Professor of Obstetrics and Gynecology, The Mount Sinai School of Medicine; Former Clinical Professor of Obstetrics and Gynecology, Columbia University College of Physicians and Surgeons; Former Lecturer, Harvard School of Public Health; Chairman, Medical Committee, International Planned Parenthood Federation."[75]

Guttmacher punctuated his advice to women with references to his own authority and to the authority of his profession in general. In one section of his book he wrote, "Very likely there is a small but real danger from using the pill. However, the risk is so slight and the advantages of effectiveness and acceptability so great that for most patients, it is a risk worth taking. Since I am the physician President of Planned Parenthood, I probably have the biggest pill practice in the world. . . . And I advise the pill for members of my own family." Guttmacher warned women not to believe what they might read, "particularly in women's magazines." He wrote, "Many other medical charges have been made against oral contraceptives, particularly in women's magazines. Certainly an unsubstantiated medical scare story or a distorted report consisting of half-truths will often capture a reader's interest more than just the facts."[76]

At the end of his book Guttmacher included a section in which he reviewed questions patients ask most frequently about birth control. In response to the question, "Is birth control harmful?" this physician, who had earlier insensitively explained that the opening of a woman's cervix was approximately "the size of a knitting needle," offered women only these "facts" about oral contraceptives:

> No—absolutely not, for more than 99 out of a hundred users. The only known exceptions occur very rarely among users of the pill. . . . Birth control has been recognized as an important part of medical care by numerous professional organizations, including the American Medical Association, the American Public Health Association, the New York Academy of Medicine, and many specialists' groups and state and county medical societies. Contraceptive products are advertised in medical journals and have to be passed by the U.S. Food and Drug Administration before they can be sold. Whether you hold the medical profession in high or low esteem, you would have to be paranoid to believe that the overwhelming majority of American doctors would endorse—and prescribe—a medical technique if there were any serious questions as to its safety.[77]

Paranoid or not, many women, and some physicians, had questions about the safety of the pill that they considered serious enough to warrant a search for an alternative method of birth control.

2 The Dalkon Shield Story

D r. Hugh J. Davis, Director of the Family Planning Clinic at Johns Hopkins University, was among many physicians who began to design and experiment with new models of intrauterine devices in the 1960s. Davis designed a closed ring device which he called the "Incon Ring." The shape of that device was the precursor of the "improved" model that came to be called the Dalkon Shield.[1]

In 1968 Davis was a partner in a firm called Lerner Laboratories with an electrical engineer, Irwin Lerner, and an attorney, Robert E. Cohn. Lerner is credited with having "invented" the Dalkon Shield by adding a central membrane and lateral spikes to the frame of the Incon Ring.[2] A close inspection of a Dalkon Shield reveals a ring shaped exactly like the Incon surrounding the central membrane. The patent for this device was obtained in Lerner's name. Davis held the patent for the Incon Ring but was required to assign his financial interest in that device to Johns Hopkins. Because the patent for the shield was in Lerner's name alone, Davis did not have to assign his interest in it to the university. Davis began testing the new device at Johns Hopkins in 1968. In 1969 Davis, Lerner, and Cohn formed the Dalkon Corporation and named the shield device, previously called the D Shield, the Dalkon Shield.[3]

In 1967, the year before Davis began to test the shield, the U.S. Food and Drug Administration directed Dr. Roger B. Scott to conduct a survey of the Fellows of the American College of Obstetricians and Gynecologists to discover the incidence of deaths and critical illnesses associated with the use of intrauterine devices by women in the United States. Ten deaths were reported, all caused by sequelae of pelvic infections. The women who died ranged in age from 20 to 42 years. Seven of these women had used the Lippes Loop; two used a coil device; one IUD was not identified by brand. The pathogens identified as responsible for the infections included gonorrhea (one case); E-coli (one case); streptococci (four cases); and four cases of unspecified infectious organisms.[4] One hundred ninety-two cases of nonfatal critical illness were also reported, and there were fifteen uterine perforations. The perforating devices named were twelve bow-shaped devices and one Incon Ring; two were not identified.

In its January 1968 report the FDA's Advisory Committee on Obstetrics and Gynecology recommended that sterile precautions be used during insertion of all IUDs, and called for increased research support for the development of more efficient and medically safer IUD products and insertion procedures. The committee reported that IUDs were efficient in preventing pregnancy, but less so than oral contraceptives. They advised against the continued use of closed devices like the Incon Ring because those devices were responsible for "intestinal obstruction in a disproportionately large number of cases" when perforation occurred.[5]

Scott published the results of his survey in *Obstetrics and Gynecology* in March 1968. The same month two other physicians published a study of 708 Lippes Loops and two Marguilies Permaspirals that had been inserted into "the 710 women who chose intrauterine contraception between July 1, 1964 and July 31, 1965" at the University of Michigan Medical School. Twenty-five of the women had become pregnant, five of them with ectopic pregnancies. Eleven developed pelvic infections, including four who required hospitalization. One woman suffered a tubo-ovarian abscess. Two of the eleven women with infections tested positive for gonorrhea; the other nine infections were listed as nonspecific in origin. Three women suffered perforations. Only 49 percent of the women continued to use the method by June 1967, and among those women 25 percent reported "continuing alteration in menstrual function or other symptoms."[6]

In June 1968 Ledger and Schrader reported the death from septicemia of a twenty-six-year-old mother of four children. Three days after having a Lippes Loop inserted, the woman became critically ill and was hospitalized. A hysterectomy was performed because of the severity of the infection. Nine hours later, "bleeding from her mouth, vagina and rectum,"[7] she died. In the same issue with Ledger and Schrader's report, Charles H. Birnberg, creator of the IUD known as the Birnberg Bow, extolled the "great advantages" of the intrauterine device and urged continuing development of the method "to reach full effectiveness." Birnberg listed the following advantages of intrauterine devices: "Use of an IUD requires but a single decision on the part of the woman. . . . the male is not required to participate in the method. . . . the devices are inexpensive. . . . they are phenomenally effective . . . and they are safe when properly inserted and managed."[8]

The next month George Solish and Gregory Majzlin reported the development of a new stainless steel spring for intrauterine contraception. The device was Majzlin's own Majzlin Spring. While admitting that experience with the device was "still meager," the authors claimed "promising results," particularly with insertions "in 7 nulliparous private patients." The authors believed the lack of side effects in those patients suggested that the spring might be "more acceptable to the nulligravida than other IUDs have been." They believed that the "low level of motivation demanded" by the general method made IUD use "particularly attractive." The additional advantages of the spring, in their opinion, were that it was relatively inert; it retained its shape indefinitely; it was preloaded into its own disposable inserter and then sealed into a sterile package; the method of insertion helped to bring about "more exact placement of the device in the uterine fundus"; and the device was flexible and would therefore adapt itself "to the configuration of the uterine cavity." These features made the new device competitive with other IUDs, according to the authors, who said it had been "developed in an attempt to correct some of the apparent shortcomings of IUDs already in use." The article did not disclose any commercial interest that either of the authors might have had in the device's sale.[9]

In December 1968 Mogens Osler and Paul Lebech wrote about another new device called an Antigon. They reported no perforations, eighteen pregnancies, fifty-six expulsions, and twenty-two removals among 707 patients during a one-year trial period in Copenhagen. A note at the end of the article announced that the device was being modified because of reports that closed devices were, "in a few cases," associated with "intestinal strangulation following perforation." Lebech was one of the inventors of the Antigon.[10] As in most articles about IUDs written by their inventors, Lebech's interest in the device was not disclosed.

In May 1969 an article praising IUDs appeared in the *New England Journal of Medicine*. Published in the "Medical Intelligence" section of the journal, the article claimed that "the availability of antibiotics has given the physician a means of treating the most common serious adverse effect, infection." The author identified other major advantages as "a minimal need for patient motivation, the lack of known systemic effects, few problems with either distribution of the device or continued patient use, and the negligible nonrecurring expense."[11]

In August 1969 Dhall, Dhall, and Gupta reported eight cases of perforation in women wearing the Lippes Loop. Four devices were listed as partial perforations because the loops were found still poking through the uterine tissue. The other four devices had pushed all the way through the uterus to reach the peritoneal cavity.[12] The next month H. Robert Misenhimer and Rafael Garcia-Bunuel reported two deaths in infants born of women whose IUDs had been retained during their pregnancies. One infant died twenty-nine hours after birth; the other lived for 114 hours. The IUDs worn by the two women were not identified. Each infant died of fungal infections.[13]

In December 1969 Jaime Zipper et al. reported on the addition of metallic copper to the T device. They wrote, "By adding metallic copper to an inert device a new and promising avenue of contraceptive development has been opened." One of the authors, Howard J. Tatum, who later became an outspoken critic of the Dalkon Shield, was the inventor of the original T device; Tatum and Zipper invented the Copper T. Any commercial interest that authors Tatum or Zipper might have had in the promotion of their device was not disclosed in their report.[14]

Dr. Hugh J. Davis, inventor of the Incon Ring and partner in the Dalkon Corporation, testified at the 1970 Senate hearings on oral contraceptives. He claimed that the effectiveness of the pill had been "greatly overrated."[15] Davis stressed that the effects of other methods of contraception, including the IUD, were local and not systemic. He complained that "very little research and development money has been allocated to developing safer local alternatives." Of the alternative methods available, Davis claimed the IUD was most effective. He said, "In our experience, some modern intrauterine devices provide a 99 percent protection against pregnancy."[16]

Senator Thomas J. McIntyre asked Davis, "I understand that you yourself have devised an intrauterine device that is extremely good?" Davis answered, "This is not a development of mine. We have been testing a whole series of intrauterine devices for the last seven years and the particular device we have been using for the last 18 months has proven quite effective." As to the potential hazards of IUD use, Davis testified, "I think that you can safely state that the major hazards of the use of an intrauterine device are related to the technical act of insertion, and that if you carry out technical precautions, it carries less risk than a smallpox vaccination which can under unusual circumstances lead to meningitis and death."[17]

Attorney James P. Duffy III raised the question of Dr. Davis' financial interest in promoting the use of IUDs. He said, "Doctor, while we're on the subject of intrauterine devices, in our preparation for these hearings we became aware of the report that indicated that you had recently patented such a device. Is there any truth to that report?" Davis replied, "I hold no recent patent on any intrauterine device." Davis explained that his name appeared "on a joint patent together with a Mr. Jones, and this patent is held jointly by the Johns Hopkins University." However, Davis explained, "That particular device was a ring which was used for experimental purposes and has never been marketed and I doubt ever will be marketed." Mr. Duffy asked, "Then you have no particular commercial interest in any of the intrauterine devices?" Davis answered, "That is correct."[18]

Just a week after Davis testified at the Senate hearings, his article "The Shield Intrauterine Device: A Superior Modern Contraceptive" appeared in the *American Journal of Obstetrics and Gynecology*. In it he claimed that "trials of intrauterine devices in more than 5,000 women have been underway at our institution. . . . Recent experiences with a shield design approaches [*sic*] the ideal of combining very low pregnancy rates with minimal side effects." Davis reported a pregnancy rate of 1.1 percent in "the first year of experience with the Dalkon Shield at Johns Hopkins." He described the shield as a "light and flexible" device with "a central membrane . . . precluding bowel strangulation in the event of perforation," and asserted that the shield was both more effective in preventing pregnancy than sequential oral contraceptives and had the added advantage of being "a modern IUD without the actual or potential hazards of systemic medication for birth control."[19]

In May 1970 the "Medical News" section of the *Journal of the American Medical Association* carried an article entitled "Virtually Failsafe IUD Seen in Year." The article reported, "Within a year we should have an intrauterine contraceptive device with a pregnancy rate of 0.5 percent or less, reports Hugh J. Davis, M.D." The next month the A. H. Robins Corporation purchased the Dalkon Shield from the Dalkon Corporation. The Dalkon Corporation received $750,000, plus 10 percent royalties. According to Morton Mintz, Davis was paid $242,812.50 for his share of the initial proceeds. Davis, Lerner, and another stockholder of the Dalkon Corporation, Thad Earl, were hired by A. H. Robins as consultants.[20]

In the days immediately preceding the purchase, A. H. Robins was warned by several of its own top executives of potential problems with the Dalkon Shield. A. H. Robins vice president Fred A. Clark discovered discrepancies in the pregnancy rates quoted by Davis in his original study, and wrote a memo to that effect. The day before the purchase, another vice president at Robins recommended "continuing research" because of the recent addition of copper to the Dalkon Shield and the inadequate follow-up of patients in Davis' original study. Corporate officials were clearly aware that a higher pregnancy rate had been found when women who participated in the study were followed for a couple of months after the study ended, and they knew that no studies had been done since copper had been added to the device. But the recommendations for continuing research were ignored, and A. H. Robins continued to cite Davis' original results as accurate and applicable to the modified device.[21]

In September 1970 Davis coauthored "Mechanisms of Action of In-

trauterine Contraceptives in Women" with Dr. John Lesinski. In the article the authors claimed, "Further improvements in IUD performance
will be forthcoming shortly. Modern devices already approach an ideal
contraceptive. They are effective, medically safe and have few side effects. We are confident that these superior qualities will increasingly
make intrauterine devices a first-choice method in the clinical practice
of contraception." They noted that the "strictly local mechanisms which
prevent conception without producing widespread systemic effects"
made IUDs "an ideal contraceptive." They also claimed that the local
mechanisms were enhanced by maximum contact between the IUD's
surface and the endometrium. In addition, they maintained that "certain types of plastic," for example, polypropylene, the material used in
the Dalkon Shield, "are apparently more effective in inducing appropriate endometrial responses than others."[22]

In October 1970 the A. H. Robins Corporation modified the shape
and content of the Dalkon Shield. Barium sulfate was added to increase
the visibility of the device in X-rays. The central plastic membrane was
made thinner; the ends of the spikes were rounded; and the plastic rim
to which the string was tied was thickened. The shield had changed considerably since Davis had conducted the initial tests at Johns Hopkins in
1968, and in December 1970 A. H. Robins began a "ten investigator
study" scheduled to last five years. A month later the Dalkon Shield was
released for sale. An aggressive marketing campaign accompanied the
release. Although follow-up of Davis' original test group two months
after he completed his initial study showed a pregnancy rate of approximately 6 percent, the marketing campaign used Davis' original figure,
1.1 percent. No mention was made of the untested structural alterations
to the device. A new size Dalkon Shield was marketed for women who
had never been pregnant. That size had also never been tested, but that
fact was not made public. Neither health care providers nor their clients
could have known that Davis had a financial interest in the Dalkon
Shield; nor were they informed that he had been retained as a paid consultant for the firm. According to the National Women's Health Network, A. H. Robins distributed to prospective clients 199,000 reprints

of Davis' article "The Shield Intrauterine Device: A Superior Modern Contraceptive."[23]

According to one report there were "over 70 IUD models" available by March 1971. The manufacturers of new devices faced competition with other contraceptive products and with other models of IUDs. Oral contraceptives claimed the largest share of the market for all birth control products, and the Lippes Loop was the most widely used IUD when A. H. Robins began its promotion of the Dalkon Shield. The corporation claimed that its new product was "superior to the pill." It was allegedly more effective than sequential pills, and it produced a local, not a systemic, contraceptive effect. Unlike the oral contraceptives, the IUD did not cause weight gain, depression, or backache, according to the manufacturer. The corporation also claimed that the shield was superior to other brands of intrauterine devices. It supposedly had the lowest pregnancy rate, and it boasted a "superior design" that was supposed to reduce expulsions, cramping, and bleeding, leading to "exceptional patient tolerance."[24]

Despite these features, the corporation began receiving complaints from physicians as early as one month after sales began. One physician wrote saying that he had "ordered all shields out" of his office. He had inserted "thousands" of IUDs of other types without encountering problems with the procedure, but after inserting ten Dalkon Shields he said that he "found the procedure to be the most traumatic manipulation ever perpetrated on womankind."[25]

In 1971 Davis, then a salaried consultant for A. H. Robins, published *Intrauterine Devices for Contraception: The IUD*. Although called a textbook, this publication read like a promotional tract for the Dalkon Shield. Davis dedicated the book "to Reverend Thomas Malthus, who discovered the problem before the world understood the remedy and Dr. Richard Richter, who discovered the remedy before the world understood the problem." The problem discovered by Malthus was overpopulation; the remedy Davis credited to Richter was the intrauterine device. The best remedy of all, according to Davis, was the Dalkon Shield.

In his first two chapters Davis discussed the history of intrauterine devices and demographic considerations for their use. Davis claimed, "We [are] losing the population war globally," and said, "Experience in the decade 1960 to 1970 in dealing with population pressures indicates that the most successful programs have emphasized the use of intra-uterine devices, medical abortions, and sterilizations." He concluded that "balanced national and international programs" were needed "so that the quality of life may indeed be preserved by the prevention of excessive human life."[26]

After explaining the global "need" for intrauterine devices in general, Davis set out to compare different models of IUDs. First he discussed the "mechanisms of action" that allegedly enhanced IUD effectiveness. Two factors were important: the surface area of the IUD in contact with the endometrium, and the "chemotactic response" caused by the materials used in the device. According to Davis, the devices with the greatest surface area yielded the lowest pregnancy rates, and the materials poly-ethylene and copper enhanced the "anti-conceptive effect." Among the IUDs he reviewed, he found that the "copper shield" yielded the most promising results.[27]

Davis' reference to the Dalkon Shield as a "copper shield" and his assertion that the copper had an "anti-conceptive effect" eventually became sources of contention between Davis and A. H. Robins. When the Dalkon Shield was marketed, the FDA classified "inert" IUDs as devices, but IUDs containing "active" materials that contributed to their efficacy were considered drugs. Drugs were subject to stricter regulation than devices. To prevent the Dalkon Shield from being classified as a drug, the corporation insisted that the copper in the Dalkon Shield was there only to strengthen it, arguing that there was too little copper in the Dalkon Shield for it to have any biologic effect. Davis, however, cited the addition of copper as a factor enhancing the superior ability of the Dalkon Shield to prevent pregnancy. Ultimately the corporation was able to convince the FDA that the Dalkon Shield was a device. The corporation was then able to market the product without the extensive prior testing that would have been required if it had been classified as a drug.[28]

After asserting that the Dalkon Shield was superior to other IUDs by virtue of its mechanisms of action, Davis returned to a defense of IUDs in general, comparing the IUD to oral contraceptives. Davis claimed that the pill was more effective when used perfectly by highly motivated contraceptors, but that the IUD was still highly effective and required little motivation. The pill, Davis said, had "widespread systematic effects" which made its long-term use in the absence of a "medical indication for the use of ovulatory suppressants" inadvisable, particularly given "the availability of excellent alternatives." As an "excellent alternative," according to him, the IUD offered "local protection; secure protection; convenient protection; safe protection; and prolonged protection." Davis devoted one chapter to a discussion of IUD insertion and removal procedures. He listed five contraindications to IUD use: "known or suspected uterine pregnancy; acute or subacute pelvic inflammatory disease; a history of incapacitating dysmenorrhea or menorrhagia; known or suspected cervical or uterine neoplasia; and hypoplasia, stenosis or distortion of the cavity." In addition to careful selection of patients, Davis discouraged the use of devices that embed in the endometrium (bow, spring, open ring, coil, and loop devices) and the use of devices made of poor quality plastic.[29]

Davis stressed the importance of professional competence in inserting intrauterine devices. He recommended routine use of an instrument to determine the size, shape, and position of the uterine cavity. He advised that a tenaculum be used to hold the cervix and provide traction in order to assure proper placement of the device and to guard against perforation. He suggested the use of anesthesia to reduce pain. With "strict adherence to a sound management protocol," he claimed, "untoward complications" could be "largely eliminated."[30] (This emphasis on the importance of professional competence would be relied on later by A. H. Robins in its attempts to blame physicians for the complications that women suffered from the Dalkon Shield.)

Davis entitled his next chapter, "Choice of Device." He compared a variety of intrauterine devices with charts and graphs that purported to measure rates of effectiveness, expulsions, and medical removals. The "shield type of IUD" was superior on all counts. It was better tolerated by women who had never been pregnant; its effectiveness surpassed its nearest competitor two to one; it was expelled less often than any other IUD; and its rate of removal for medical reasons was 2 percent, compared to a 15 percent removal rate in users of the nearest competitor on this score, the Lippes Loop. One chart in this chapter was "Performance of Major IUDs Developed since 1930." Davis compared twenty-three devices, giving "Percent Complications on Three Counts: Pregnancy Rates, Expulsion Rates and Medical Removals." He did not consider length of time or prevalence of usage for any of the devices; some were new, others were old and had been used for a short time long ago, and some had been used extensively for many years. The Dalkon Shield—one of the newest devices compared—showed an overall complication rate of less than 5 percent. Its closest competitor was the Heart device, with approximately 8 percent complications. The most dismal showings were with the Small Spiral (50 percent) and the Lippes Loop (42 percent). All sizes of the Lippes Loop, which was the most widely used intrauterine device at that time, had more complications than the infamous Grafenberg Ring, a silk device that had been linked to massive pelvic infections when it was used in the 1930s, and had caused physicians to be skeptical of IUDs for three decades. Only seven of the twenty-three devices, all of them relatively new at the time, scored better than the Grafenberg Ring. One device, the Spring Coil, which was shown to have an overall complication rate of 33 percent, surpassed all the others in effectiveness, with an incredible pregnancy rate of zero percent. The Dalkon Shield fared best in the category of medical removals, showing approximately one-sixth the rate of its nearest competitor. The Majzlin Spring and the M device showed slightly lower expulsion rates than the Dalkon Shield but dramatically higher rates of medical removals. The Heart showed a lower pregnancy rate, but higher rates of both expulsion and medical removal. Pregnancy rates with the Dalkon Shield were comparable to the M device and the Saf-T-Coil, each of which had double the overall complication rate attributed to the shield.[31]

In a chapter devoted to ethical considerations, Davis again pleaded for the acceptance of IUDs in general, this time directing his arguments to theologians. He argued that IUDs prevented conception without causing abortions: "The sine qua non of conception is implantation of a viable ovum, and the biologic integrity of the ovum can only be demonstrated by competent implantation. Prior to the critical event of successful implantation, every woman is potentially pregnant, but pregnancy cannot be said to exist because the process of conception is incomplete."[32]

In discussing septic complications, Davis maintained that "unless a documented febrile illness follows immediately on the heels of the insertion procedure a cause-effect relationship with the IUD is unlikely." Because he presumed all later infections to be unrelated to the IUD's presence, he excluded reports of such illnesses in the assessment of IUD complications. Davis blamed all IUD-related infections on improper "manufacture, packaging, patient preparation and insertion." According to him, "The routine use of sterile, pre-packaged devices and aseptic insertion technique could unquestionably reduce the incidence of septic complications associated with IUD insertion."[33]

In illustrated appendixes Davis compared thirty-two intrauterine devices. The Dalkon Shield again showed the most favorable overall performance record when pregnancy, expulsion, and removal rates were considered together. Davis listed the inventor of each IUD shown, crediting Irwin Lerner as the inventor of the Dalkon Shield. Nowhere in the book did Davis acknowledge his financial interest in the "superior modern IUD" he praised. Years later, however, in a deposition given to plaintiff's attorney, Bradley Post, Davis acknowledged that the A. H. Robins Corporation had read the manuscript before it was published and had paid for the illustrations.[34]

The same month that Davis' book was released, A. H. Robins began a two-year study of the Dalkon Shield using baboons. According to the National Women's Health Network, 12.5 percent of the baboon subjects died during the experiment; 30 percent suffered uterine perforations.[35]

Howard J. Tatum, inventor of the T device and coinventor of the Copper T, published an article in April 1972 giving an "evolutionary" history of intrauterine devices. In it he lamented the "conservatism" that he said had impeded development. Tatum wrote, "Much of the criticism which was directed toward Grafenberg and against the intrauterine ring was based more upon the conservative traditionalism of the gynecologist than upon scientifically valid reasons. It was indeed a tragedy that conservatism prevailed since the traditional taboo against inserting a foreign body into the uterine cavity thwarted the advance of contraceptive technology for at least 30 years."[36]

Tatum was concerned about a particular aspect of the "traditional taboo": the idea that "the infected or potentially infected endometrial cavity . . . could not be invaded safely by instruments and certainly should not immediately receive an intrauterine foreign body to serve as a contraceptive device." Referring to this traditional concept as "dogma," he claimed that it was "no longer tenable under most circumstances." Tatum helped organize an international program supported by the Population Council. He explained, "A double blind study was set up . . . to answer the question, 'can an intrauterine contraceptive be safely and effectively introduced into the infected uterus immediately following curettage or ovum evacuation for an incomplete abortion?'" He added, "The only patients who were excluded from the study were those who had fulminating peritonitis." By Tatum's assessment, the results of the study confirmed his suspicion that traditional dogma did not "pertain to modern medicine."[37]

In the next few months new information began to challenge Davis' and Tatum's arguments. First, in April, Dr. Mary Gabrielson addressed a meeting of the American Association of Planned Parenthood Physicians in Detroit. She presented her findings from a study of two Planned Parenthood clinics in California. The pregnancy rate among the women she studied reached four to five times the rate published by Davis and used by A. H. Robins in advertising. Gabrielson also reported a medical removal rate of 25 percent and an infection rate of 5 percent. Second, in May, the *Journal of the American Medical Association* printed "A Simple Way to Remove IUDs after Perforation." Dr. John Leventhal of Harvard reported a method he and his colleagues had used to remove thirteen Lippes Loops and three Dalkon Shields that had perforated women's uteri. Leventhal observed, "The loop appears to be associated far less frequently with an interperitoneal reaction" than the Dalkon Shield. Then, in June, Thad Earl, one of the four partners in the Dalkon Corporation when the Dalkon Shield was sold to A. H. Robins, wrote a letter to A. H. Robins saying that some of his patients had become pregnant with the shield in place. When the shield was left in place, the women aborted spontaneously "at three and a half to five months." Earl wrote, "In my [*sic*] six pregnancies I removed one and she carried full term, the rest all aborted and became septic. . . . I realize that this is a small statistic but . . . most men [*sic*] are experiencing the same problem."[38]

Sales of the Dalkon Shield increased from 1971 to 1972, but began to decline by the middle of 1972.[39] In September 1972 Davis published "Intrauterine Contraceptive Devices: Present Status and Future Prospects." In that article, he blamed confusion for the delay in acceptance of IUDs by the medical profession. He said that the use of IUDs had "remained outside the pale of respectable gynecologic practice until the past decade" because "true intrauterine contraceptive devices" had been confused with "the stem pessaries inserted by quacks and granny midwives to provoke abortion at the turn of the century." Echoing Tatum's sentiments, Davis attributed a "general reluctance to insert any foreign material into the uterine cavity" to prejudice on the part of physicians. He said, "Experience with the IUD technique in numerous clinical studies has shown that most such prejudice against the method has been unwarranted," and he repeated his argument that pelvic infections coincident with IUD use were not attributable to the devices unless they occurred immediately following insertion. Davis claimed that pelvic inflammatory disease was "seldom encountered" in "private patients fitted with intrauterine devices," adding, "Pelvic infections observed months or years following IUD insertion are usually coincidental in nature, responding in the usual fashion to antibiotic therapy without removal of the device."[40]

Davis again found fault with coils, bows, springs, loops, spirals, and ring devices. He stated that the T device held promise and included it with the shield as a "second generation IUD." He said it was "a striking improvement" over "the prototype rings, coils and loops." But the shield remained, in his opinion, "the most effective of the commercially available devices." Davis cautioned that "in situations demanding virtually absolute protection against pregnancy" patients should be advised to use contraceptive foam along with the IUD. He claimed that the IUD was more effective than sequential birth control pills, but that even "the best result . . . published with a commercially available IUD" was 99— not 100—percent effective. Investigators learned much later that Davis had recommended the use of contraceptive foam to women who participated in his initial tests of the Dalkon Shield at Johns Hopkins. This may have been one factor explaining the very low pregnancy rates reported at the close of that study. Neither health and family planning personnel nor women who would use the Dalkon Shield were informed of this recommendation when the Dalkon Shield went on the market in January 1971.[41]

A. H. Robins made two changes in promotional materials during 1972. They removed the claim that the Dalkon Shield could easily be inserted without anesthesia from their advertisements to physicians; and they changed the patient brochure, adding the assurance to women that if pregnancy should accidentally occur with the Dalkon Shield in place, no harm would come to woman or fetus. The device, they said, would simply be moved "gently aside" by the amniotic sac.[42]

By the end of 1972 A. H. Robins had launched a second massive advertising campaign in the United States and had expanded exports. Largely through the U.S. Agency for International Development (AID), the corporation shipped approximately two million Dalkon Shields to seventy-nine other countries by 1975. Some of those Dalkon Shields were sold to AID at a 48 percent discount. They were shipped unsterilized, with one inserter for every ten shields and one set of instructions for every thousand.[43] In the United States, where thousands of cases of pelvic infection associated with the Dalkon Shield have been documented, the devices were sold in individualized sterile packets with disposable inserters. No estimates of the comparative rates of infection between women who received presterilized Dalkon Shields and women who received them shipped in bulk are available.

In January 1973 Arnold Sprague and Van Jenkins reported three cases of uterine perforation with the Dalkon Shield. One woman was twenty-four years old. Her Dalkon Shield was found "embedded in the anterior of the uterus." An ectopic pregnancy was suspected. The physicians performed "a total abdominal hysterectomy and bilateral salpingectomy," but found no ectopic pregnancy. The other two women were pregnant. One had an unruptured ectopic pregnancy, and a left salpingectomy and oophorectomy were performed. The other woman had her Dalkon Shield surgically removed along with her appendix. Her pregnancy had progressed into the fifth month and the woman "continued to do well" when the article was written.[44]

Bernard Draper and Eugene White published an article critical of the Dalkon Shield in the same issue with the Sprague and Jenkins article. Draper and White wrote, "The Dalkon Shield intrauterine device has been reported as a highly effective 'second generation' intrauterine contraceptive. It has received wide publicity and popularity in the mass media. Our experience with the device is reviewed because of an unexpected apparent high failure rate." The authors reported seven pregnancies among 167 patients, most in association with postpartum insertions.[45]

The same month Byrne Marshall, James Hepler, and Masaharu Jinguji reported a case of fatal streptococcus pyogenes septicemia. They wrote, "A previously healthy 29 year old woman . . . four months after her Dalkon Shield was inserted . . . died of septic shock 63 hours after the onset of her illness. . . . The admitting diagnosis was acute pelvic inflammatory disease . . . autopsy revealed acute salpingitis and endometritis . . . in addition to diffuse peritonitis." The authors noted that such deaths usually occur "within 72 hours after the onset of infection," making any delay in diagnosis very likely to result in death.[46]

In May 1973 the Food and Drug Administration seized 9,000 Majzlin Spring intrauterine devices and ordered that sales of that device be immediately stopped. The Majzlin Spring had been marketed since 1968, and "tens of thousands" were allegedly inserted into women's bodies during the five years that it was sold. The FDA had received complaints about the device as early as 1970. Physicians said the devices tended to embed in the endometrium, push through the myometrium, and ulti-mately work their way through the uterus. On May 25, 1973, a House government operations subcommittee convened to hear testimony from representatives of the FDA about the regulation of intrauterine devices. The three-year delay in halting the distribution of Majzlin Springs after they were known to cause serious, even fatal, complications was a subject of concern to the committee. An FDA representative explained that the Administration's policy was to evaluate the risks associated with IUDs in relation to the expected benefits. Action was taken to stop the sale of Majzlin Springs once the FDA officials were convinced that its benefits no longer outweighed the risk to individuals.[47]

In July 1973 R. W. Jones, A. Parker, and Max Elstein reported their experiences with the Dalkon Shield in the *British Medical Journal.* Claim-ing a 98 percent follow-up among 377 women over a period of seventeen months, the authors found a 4.7 percent pregnancy rate. This they be-lieved was similar to the rate for the Lippes Loop, but they found a lower expulsion rate with the shield. They concluded that "the shield is an advance in intrauterine contraception but . . . the complication rate quoted by Davis is an under-estimation."[48] The article did not mention any relationship between the authors and A. H. Robins, although Mor-ton Mintz lists Elstein as one of Robins' paid British consultants. Elstein eventually became an "expert witness" testifying on behalf of Robins in a Dalkon Shield trial in St. Paul, Minnesota.[49]

In August 1973 Donald R. Ostergard, another paid consultant for A. H. Robins and a member of their ten-investigator team, published "Intrauterine Contraception in Nulliparas with the Dalkon Shield." Os-tergard wrote, "Intrauterine contraception usually is not offered to nul-liparous patients because 'first generation' devices proved unreliable for this group of patients. Recently, experience with a 'second generation' device, the Dalkon Shield, contradicts this experience."[50]

In October 1973 John Esposito, Donald Zaron, and George Zaron published "A Dalkon Shield Embedded in a Myoma: Case Report of an Unusual Displacement of an Intrauterine Contraceptive Device." The authors stated that they had previously reported "that perforation only takes place at the time of insertion." They had changed their minds about this, claiming that "there are two types of perforations, the immediate traumatic perforation, and a later perforation caused by gradual erosion of the uterine musculature." They complained that the Dalkon Shield was difficult to locate with X rays because "its degree of opacity . . . was not adequate for visualization."[51]

In the same month Dr. W. H. Harris reported two cases of uterine perforation, one with a Dalkon Shield and the other with a Lippes Loop. In each of the women the IUD strings remained visible, extending through the cervix and into the vagina in their normal position even after perforation. It had previously been believed that the visibility of the strings assured that the IUD was in place within the uterus. Perforation was suspected only when the strings were no longer visible.[52]

Questions about the safety of intrauterine devices began to appear in the mass media after the FDA's seizure of Majzlin Springs. *Good Housekeeping* published an article entitled "Are IUD Contraceptives Safe?" reporting that "more than 3,000,000 women" in the United States were wearing IUDs. The FDA had removed the Majzlin Spring from the market, the article claimed, "because studies show that complications, such as cramps, bleeding and uterine perforation, increased the longer the device was in a woman's uterus." The article did not say how many perforations were estimated to have occurred, nor did it mention any potential sequelae of uterine perforation. *Good Housekeeping* reported that two physicians had testified at the House subcommittee hearings that adverse reaction to IUDs had been underreported, and that manufacturers' claims about IUD performance were inaccurate. The magazine did not name specific manufacturers or specific devices, except for the Majzlin Spring. It did report, however, that "spokesmen for organizations such as Planned Parenthood Federation of America and the American College of Obstetricians and Gynecologists quickly responded to these criticisms defending the IUD as both safe and effective when used for properly selected individuals." *Good Housekeeping* reporters "interviewed authorities around the country." One such authority was Dr. Louise B. Tyler, director of the family planning division of the American

College of Obstetricians and Gynecologists. Tyler said, "Serious infection is very rare . . . and has been reduced in the past two or three
years. . . . The majority of infections that do occur now are mild and can
usually be treated successfully without removing the IUD." The authors
also interviewed Dr. Alan Guttmacher, president of the Planned Parenthood Federation of America, who assured readers, "For most women, it
is an acceptable and effective method of contraception when prescribed,
inserted, and managed under competent medical supervision and with
disclosure of information to the patient."[53]

A similar article in *McCall's* the next month stated, "IUDs are less
reliable in preventing pregnancy than the two-hormone pill. . . . Among
their real hazards are pelvic infections and perforations of the uterus.
Both problems rarely occur if the woman has had a thorough medical
exam beforehand."[54]

In the Boston Women's Health Collective's *Our Bodies, Ourselves,* the
section on intrauterine contraception mentioned the Dalkon Shield specifically: "The Dalkon Shield is the most recent hope of never-pregnant
women. In its first year and a half of wide usage the Shield seems to have
low expulsion and complication rates, but its pregnancy rate in women
who have never been pregnant seems to be higher than expected. So
there is no perfect IUD." The section included the following warning
about infection with IUDs in general: "Infection flares up after insertion
if the doctor does not maintain sterile conditions or if you have gonorrhea, severe vaginal infection, or pelvic inflammatory disease at the time
of insertion. . . . While you have an IUD in place you run about a five
percent chance of infection in vagina, uterus, tubes, ovaries (according
to one Boston doctor)." But the book also offered reassurance, saying, "If
you get pregnant with the IUD in place and go on with the pregnancy,
there is no danger to the infant. . . . At least the effects of the IUD are
local—if something goes wrong your uterus hurts and you seek medical
help. . . . Chances of becoming pregnant [after the IUD is removed] are
the same as before using the IUD."[55]

In February 1974 *Good Housekeeping* described the IUD as "a small flexible plastic or metal device" that was "growing in popularity." A chart

listed "Irregular bleeding, spotting, cramps and discomfort" as "common early side effects." "Pelvic inflammatory disease (infection) and perforation of the uterus" were listed as "rare and potentially dangerous side effects." The article stated that "a major advantage is that once an IUD is inserted, no further action by the woman is required except for regular checks that she herself can make to be certain the IUD is in place."[56]

In March 1974 Dr. Johanna Perlmutter reported her professional experience with the Dalkon Shield. She wrote, "A pregnancy rate of 10.1 per 100 women-years was obtained . . . with no apparent reduction with time over a two-year interval. This device appears to offer no benefit as a contraceptive agent over other currently available, more effective means and cannot be recommended for continued use." In addition to the shield's high pregnancy rates, Perlmutter stated that its removal was often difficult: "In one instance it took two separate visits to the clinic and efforts by three physicians to accomplish the removal of an embedded device."[57]

The next month, L. Kent Merrill, Laurence I. Burd, and Daniel J. VerBurg reported three perforations in women using Dalkon Shields. In each case, the devices had been removed with a laparoscope from the intrapitoneal cavity. One of the women was pregnant.[58] Shortly after Merrill, Burd, and VerBurg's article appeared, J. L. Newton, Julian Elias, and Anthony Johnson wrote in the *Journal of Obstetrics and Gynecology of the British Commonwealth* that patients who were having abortions and who were "poorly motivated towards contraception" should have either a Copper 7 or a Dalkon Shield inserted. The authors recommended "immediate post-termination insertion of either the Copper 7 or Dalkon Shield as being a safe procedure, and one which helps to prevent the unnecessary suffering of a repeated unwanted pregnancy."[59]

In May 1974 physicians Robert Shine and Joseph Thompson also described their experience with the outcome of pregnancies occurring with IUDs in place: "Of the 46 pregnant patients with an in situ IUD, two had elective abortions and one was lost to follow-up. The 21 spontaneous abortions in this series represent an abortion rate of 49 percent." In addition, the authors found that "15 percent of the patients who could be followed for one year after insertion became pregnant." The women in their study had used the Lippes Loop or the Dalkon Shield. The authors found no association between pregnancy rate and type of device.[60]

Comments by several physicians followed the Shine and Thompson article. Dr. James Scott lamented that "although men have been on the moon we still don't completely understand the inside of the womb." Dr. Vivian Gibbs wrote, "I have recently had the experience of having three patients that almost died with severe infection secondary to an IUD and pregnancy. These patients required long hospitalizations, massive antibiotics, and blood transfusions. I have had many patients with lesser degrees of infection but enough to require antibiotics for treatment. I feel that there is a very definite risk to patients with an IUD." Dr. Edward Eichner blamed the incompetence of personnel inserting IUDs for the infections. He wrote, "Recently a group at Mt. Sinai (Cleveland) reported the use of IUDs inserted immediately after delivery while the patient was still on the delivery table. The follow-up has been of several years' duration. The pregnancy rate was relatively high in those inserted by the residents and the loss rate was high. The rate was very low in those inserted by qualified obstetricians and gynecologists."[61]

The *Wall Street Journal* reported on May 29, 1974, that A. H. Robins had sent a letter to physicians warning that there were "possible complications," including death, "in some women who used IUDs." According to the corporation, the problem was not unique to the Dalkon Shield. Planned Parenthood centers had decided not to continue prescribing the Dalkon Shield, the article said. The next day the *Wall Street Journal* reported further that A. H. Robins had acknowledged six maternal deaths in women who had become pregnant while using the Dalkon Shield, and "80 or 90" cases of septic abortion. Robins intended to continue marketing the device, however, claiming that there was "no reason to withdraw the product from the market."[62]

In June 1974 Dr. C. D. Christian reported five deaths—four of women wearing the Dalkon Shield and one of a woman who used a loop. The first Dalkon Shield user was thirty-one years old and had an intrauterine pregnancy of nineteen weeks' gestation. She developed "flu-like symptoms, aborted the fetus, and died within 72 hours of the onset of her first flu-like symptoms." The second was twenty-four years old and fifteen weeks pregnant. Her first symptoms involved a painful ear, a sore throat, fever, nausea, and vomiting. She aborted and died thirty-one hours after her first symptoms developed. Fewer details were given for the next two women; one woman had a loop and the other a shield. Both died after spontaneous septic abortion in the second trimester of pregnancy. The fifth woman died thirty-six hours after the onset of her symptoms. She also had a Dalkon Shield and spontaneously aborted just before she died.[63]

Christian also noted seven cases of "severely ill patients with septic abortions including six shields and one loop." He announced that he had discontinued using Dalkon Shields, "at least until further data are available." Christian said, "The greatest concern is the rather insidious yet rapid manner in which these patients became ill. In three of the five noted maternal deaths, the first symptoms, which were disarmingly innocuous, . . . occurred within thirty-one to seventy-two hours of death from sepsis and sequelae of sepsis." He also called for more attention to be given to IUD complications by the government and by physicians: "This all invites the much larger question of whether there should be more rigid evaluation and control of medical devices. Certainly, if there were five botulism deaths from one type of mushroom soup, the Food and Drug Administration would do more than put out a questionnaire." To other physicians he wrote, "We must be constantly alert to the slightest symptom or complaint. Painless dark brown spotting is common to most of the reported cases, but symptoms as apparently unrelated as sore throat, painful ear, or flu heralded the fatal sepsis in certain of the patients."[64]

At about the same time a physician wrote to the *Medical Journal of Australia* in criticism of an advertisement for the Dalkon Shield.

An advertisement in your journal was brought to my attention. This showed that the Dalkon Shield has a lower pregnancy rate, expulsion rate, and removal rate than that of other types of intrauterine contraceptive devices. . . . Closer inspection of the advertisement showed that the data presented were that of Davis who . . . was the designer of this device . . . data gathered by Snowden and Williams on United Kingdom women showed that the shield had a higher pregnancy rate . . . than that of the Lippes Loop. . . . In this world of free enterprise every company is presumably allowed to quote the evidence it feels best suits its case. Surely, however, when such contradictory evidence exists this should be considered."[65]

The letter was signed by W. G. Breed. It was followed by a reply from M. D. Reefman, medical consultant at A. H. Robins in Canterbury. He said, "Dr. Hugh J. Davis is Associate Professor of Obstetrics and Gynecology, Johns Hopkins University, Maryland, and is an early worker in the field. . . . he is not the inventor of the Dalkon Shield, but did much of the early assessment . . . and is above the commercial bias implied by your correspondent." Reefman also claimed that variance in pregnancy rates reported with the Dalkon Shield were "dependent on the insertion technique employed." Reefman quoted from four "clinical trials" in order to "further support the pregnancy rates appearing in our advertisement." He cited the "Earl Series" showing a pregnancy rate of 0.5 percent, failing to mention either Thad Earl's "commercial bias" as a stockholder in the Dalkon Corporation and a consultant of the A. H. Robins Corporation, or Earl's letter to A. H. Robins stating that he was finding an unexpectedly high rate of pregnancy, often complicated by sepsis, with the Dalkon Shield. He also cited the "Ostergard Series" showing a pregnancy rate of 1.1 percent, again failing to disclose Ostergard's relationship to A. H. Robins as a paid consultant and member of the ten-investigator study. He cited two other studies, the "Crist Series" from Norfolk, Virginia, and the "Azoury Series" published in *Lebanese Medicine*. The two latter series showed pregnancy rates of 1.4 percent and 1.2 percent, respectively.[66]

In a letter to the *British Medical Journal* the following week, J. S. Templeton, medical director at A. H. Robins in Horsham, Surrey, discussed the reports of septic abortions associated with the Dalkon Shield. He said, "Four fatalities have been reported but there is no evidence of a direct cause-and-effect relationship between the wearing of a Dalkon Shield and the occurrence of septicemia. I am certain that the apparent increase is due more to the increased number of physicians and women who prefer this method of contraception than to any inherent fault of the Dalkon Shield itself." Nevertheless, Templeton recommended that all women considering the use of a Dalkon Shield be advised that if pregnancy should occur, a therapeutic abortion "may be recommended."[67]

At the end of June 1974, A. H. Robins announced a temporary halt in sales of the Dalkon Shield in the United States, "until questions of safety are resolved." At the time the company acknowledged that seven women had died and "100 to 110" women had experienced spontaneous abortion while using the Dalkon Shield. The company made no effort to warn women wearing Dalkon Shields that "questions of safety" were unresolved.

The FDA recommended that Dalkon Shields not be used in federally funded birth control programs, but said that there was "no need for concern." In July a spokesman for the FDA announced that the agency would not recommend that Dalkon Shields be removed from the bodies of women already using them. That recommendation would not be made even if the FDA decided to ban further sales of the device. The spokesman explained that "evidence of hazards is not sufficient to warrant such a step."[68]

By August 1974, eleven fatalities and 209 septic abortions were acknowledged by A. H. Robins in association with the use of the Dalkon Shield. Debate within the FDA about whether or not the device should be banned centered on the question of relative risk. Investigators wanted to know whether the Dalkon Shield was more hazardous than other IUDs. A. H. Robins argued that it was not. Critics of the Dalkon Shield argued that its risks were exponentially greater than other IUDs'. Representatives of the FDA recommended that physicians stop inserting Dalkon Shields, but repeated their earlier recommendation that "Dalkon Shields already in place be left alone in women wearing them successfully."[69]

By October the acknowledged death toll among U.S. women using the Dalkon Shield had risen to twelve. Yet the *Wall Street Journal* published an article on the second page entitled "Robins' Dalkon Shield Found No

More Risky Than Other IUDs." Two months later the FDA gave A. H. Robins clearance to continue marketing the shield. A system of registration would be set up for all new Dalkon Shield users. (Women already wearing the Dalkon Shield were left unregistered.) The FDA also decided to develop uniform labeling for intrauterine devices.[70]

In January 1975 Dr. Russell J. Thomsen reported the death of a twenty-nine-year-old woman who had become pregnant with a Lippes Loop. The woman died a short time after delivering a stillborn infant. The cause of her death was determined to have been an amniotic fluid embolism. Thomsen reported this complication because, he said:

> A quirk of diagnostic classification . . . can lead to the conjecture that even more maternal deaths may have involved this intriguing relationship but remain unknown to the medically inquisitive person. It is a fact that the standard reference for classification of diseases used by the hospitals and agencies dealing with the collection of health data does not include adequate classification numbers for relating IUDs to associated complications. . . . the lack of coding precludes anything but a guess of the number [of major complications] experienced.[71]

Also in January, Dr. Leroy Weekes published "Complications of Intrauterine Contraceptive Devices," in which he claimed that uterine perforations sometimes resulted from improper insertion techniques. He pointed out that the visibility of the IUD strings did not necessarily indicate that no perforation had occurred, and reported that "syncope [fainting] may occur upon insertion of most rigid devices," but that no treatment was usually needed other than the provision of aromatic spirits of ammonia to revive the patient. He added, however, that he did know of one case in which a woman died of cardiac arrest while having an intrauterine device inserted.[72]

Weekes stated that "perforation of the uterine wall is one of the most serious complications of IUD insertion, especially if not noticed." Despite this, he advised physicians that it was "desirable to insert the IUD during the menstrual period when the cervical canal is most patent and when any bleeding which might be caused by the insertion is masked by the menses." He grossly understated the numbers of IUD complications

that had appeared in the literature, writing "Five mid-trimester maternal deaths and several severe cases of sepsis associated with the shield
type of intrauterine device are reported." He also seemed not to know of
the FDA's seizure of Majzlin Springs, which had occurred nearly two
years before his article appeared, going so far as to say that "newer devices such as the Majzlin Spring and Tatum T are more likely to be
tolerated since they are relatively small in size and their design allows for
easy adaptation to uterine contractions." Weekes did know of some of
the problems associated with the Dalkon Shield. He said that he had
discontinued using that device "at least until further data are available."[73]

The same month *Good Housekeeping* published another article on IUDs,
this time entitled, "Are IUDs *Really* Safe?" It reported the FDA's seizure
of Majzlin Springs and "a growing number of deaths and complications
associated with another widely used IUD, the Dalkon Shield." According to the article, the FDA had learned of 219 cases of infection and
septic abortion, including fourteen deaths, among women using the
Dalkon Shield. The report assured readers that the FDA had concluded
that the Dalkon Shield was not "significantly different from other IUDs"
and that IUDs had been "shown through extensive studies to be a safe
and reliable means of contraception when compared to other methods."
Good Housekeeping advised women to "get as much information" as possible before reaching the decision to use an IUD and added that the "skill
and experience of the specialist inserting the IUD" was related to its
"safety and effectiveness during use." The article also urged women to
support tighter regulation of intrauterine devices by the government.[74]

That same month, January 1975, A. H. Robins announced plans to
resume marketing of a modified Dalkon Shield. They planned to change
the string of the device to a monofilament type comparable to the strings
used on other IUDs. Robins' representatives claimed that they were col-
lecting unused Dalkon Shields in the United States. They said they would
notify foreign health authorities of their plan and would leave the final
decision about the collection of unused Shields in their own countries up
to those authorities.[75]

A few weeks after Robins' announcement, Dr. Howard J. Tatum and his associates reported their findings in bacteriological studies of IUD strings. They had tested strings from the Lippes Loop, the Saf-T-Coil, the Dalkon Shield, the Copper 7, and the Copper T (also known as the Tatum T). They controlled against the ascent of bacteria on the outside of the strings and tested for wicking through the interior of the strings. Only the string on the Dalkon Shield wicked. It was also the only string containing multiple filaments within a plastic sheath—the other IUDs each had monofilament strings. The results of the study had been presented to the FDA in October 1974, the same month that the FDA reported the Dalkon Shield to be "no more risky" than other IUDs.[76]

Dr. Russell Thomsen urged in a July 1975 letter to *Obstetrics and Gynecology* that other properties of the Dalkon Shield be studied in addition to the string. He wrote, "The copper content of the Dalkon Shield certainly should be considered in any plausible search for an explanation of the shield's inflammation-inducing potential."[77]

In October 1975 "The Dalkon Shield Contraceptive Device in General Practice" was published in the *Medical Journal of Australia*. The article gave the results of a follow-up study of forty-two patients. There were five pregnancies reported, including three that terminated in spontaneous abortion. One device perforated, eight were removed due to "disabling" menstrual difficulties, and two women had requested removal due to their fears "about the adverse reporting in the lay press." Twenty-two women were still wearing the device and were satisfied with it at the end of one year. Distancing himself from those promoters of IUDs whose primary motive was large-scale population control, the author commented, "The advice of the individual practitioner to his patient is on a much more personal level than that of the adviser in a demographic assault on the population explosion, and it is believed that the Dalkon Shield cannot be recommended as a desirable method of contraception control."[78]

On October 15, 1975, E. Stewart Taylor and his colleagues stated in a report, "The incidence of acute pelvic inflammatory disease is increased by the presence of an IUD, regardless of the socioeconomic status of the patient." They reported sixteen cases of tubo-ovarian abscess; nine had occurred with the Dalkon Shield, four with the Lippes Loop, one with a Saf-T-Coil, one with a spring, and one wth a "copper device." None of the women had gonorrhea, and none had a past history of pelvic inflammatory disease.[79]

Several months later, in May 1976, the *American Journal of Obstetrics and Gynecology* published a study of pelvic inflammatory disease in association with IUD use. The authors compared the percentage of infections in Dalkon Shield users with the percentage of IUD users thought to be wearing the Dalkon Shield. They wrote, "It has been estimated that the Dalkon Shield accounted for approximately 39 percent of all IUDs in use in the United States during the period of this study. Interestingly, 38 percent (10/26) of our patients with an IUD associated gynecologic infection had a Dalkon Shield in place." The authors also found that "nine out of ten patients admitted with a diagnosis of septic abortion were wearing IUDs," and that "one of every 90 admissions to the Gynecology Service was prompted by an IUD-related infection, and 27 percent of these women underwent major operations as a direct result of the infection."[80]

In the same issue Drs. Henry Kahn and Carl Tyler reported the results of their survey finding "an association between the Dalkon Shield and complicated pregnancies among women hospitalized for intrauterine contraceptive–related disorders." They stated, "Our survey data suggest that the statistical association between the standard Dalkon Shield and complicated pregnancies is observable among hospitalized women of all ages, races and geographic regions of the country."[81]

A microscopic study of the Dalkon Shield was reported in *Biomaterials, Medical Devices and Artificial Organs* in 1976. The investigators found that "the device appeared to be very poorly manufactured." They observed, "a very rough surface . . . all over the device. . . . two spicular projections . . . had a very bad surface which could form anchor sites for tissue proliferation. . . . the most surprising aspect was the thread . . . which is only composed of plasticized silk. . . . the plasticization was not uniform and some leakages appeared, providing good nidation facilities for bacteria proliferation in case of infection. When the knot was performed, neither the coating of the thread nor the plastic of the IUD was hard enough." The authors claimed that the silk used in the Dalkon Shield may have increased the contraceptive effect, because it was irritating. They added, "This kind of material could be a perfect support for bacteria." Problems with the shield, they believed, were of greater magnitude than had been suspected by those who blamed the problems solely on the string. They wrote, "Unfortunately, it is not only the plasticized string which is badly manufactured, the whole surface of the device is rough, especially where the two parts of the mold were supposed to contact each other." In the opinion of the investigators, factors contributing to infection also tended to increase the contraceptive effect, and vice versa. They said, "The question becomes: 'Could an honestly manufactured IUD which should be absolutely safe, be efficient?' The inert IUD whose configuration is the less damaging to the intrauterine cavity and the endometrium has a very questionable efficiency. Patients bearing such a device had neither bleeding nor pain. We do not completely agree with Tatum that it is only a question of surface. In our view, it is more because the endometrium was not hurt and so, it is not unsuitable for the nidation of the blastocyst."[82]

In 1976 a Medical Device Amendment gave the FDA more power to act when devices are found to be hazardous. In August of that year A. H. Robins announced that it no longer had plans to manufacture a modified Dalkon Shield. At that time, there were approximately six hundred lawsuits pending against the corporation in association with the Dalkon Shield.[83]

In December 1976 an article reporting a perforation of the large bowel by a Dalkon Shield was published in the *Journal of Reproductive Medicine* by Terry A. Athari and Cesar Pizarro. The authors estimated that the incidence of perforation with that device was one in every 387 women using it. If that estimate was accurate, nearly 12,000 women worldwide experienced that particular injury with the Dalkon Shield.[84]

Women continued to wear Dalkon Shields for many years after A. H. Robins stopped marketing them. No one knows how many women might still be wearing them. There is evidence that physicians and clinics in the United States and in many other countries continued to insert the

Dalkon Shields they had in stock long after the hazards were known. The National Women's Health Network learned of an insertion that took place in Australia in 1978. A year later the twenty-year-old woman developed pelvic inflammatory disease, which left her infertile. In 1979 Ehrenreich, Dowie, and Minkin reported in *Mother Jones* that Dalkon Shields were still being inserted in Pakistan, India, Kenya, and possibly South Africa. They also reported that the Dalkon Shield had been dispensed by physicians in Canada as late as 1977.[85]

In 1980 the A. H. Robins Corporation sent a letter to physicians advising them to remove Dalkon Shields from women still wearing them. Litigation against the company was increasing, and large settlements had been won by several claimants. Some of those settlements went to women who were injured, some went to the families of women who had died, and others to children who were injured while in utero.[86] A few settlements were for more than a million dollars; the largest was for more than six million dollars.

In April 1983 the National Women's Health Network petitioned the FDA for total recall of the Dalkon Shield from all women wearing them, with the A. H. Robins Corporation to be held responsible for all costs. In May the Department of Health and Human Services issued a news release advising that women wearing Dalkon Shields have them removed. That same month the Centers for Disease Control in Atlanta released the findings of a study showing an overall risk of pelvic inflammatory disease of 1.9 percent with all brands of IUDs, and a risk of 8.3 percent with the Dalkon Shield.[87]

In January 1984 *Contraception* published an article by Bank, MacDonald, and Wiechert "demonstrating that fluid migration occurs within and not on the surface of the multifilament tail" of the Dalkon Shield. The investigators found that "heat sealing one end of the tail prevents migration." Their findings supported a suggestion that had been made by an A. H. Robins employee in the first months after the corporation purchased the Dalkon Shield. The company rejected the employee's suggestion that they heat-seal the string, because the process would have cost several cents per device, and was therefore "too expensive" to implement.[88]

In 1984 Daniel Roberts, Douglas Horbelt, and Nola Walker published the results of electron microscopy of the multifilament Dalkon Shield. They had tested fifteen strings that had been removed from patients and found deterioration of the sheath in each one. The authors said that "deterioration of the sheath also occurs when the device is within the uterine wall or intraperitoneal. The risk of pelvic infection may be attributed to this deterioration of the sheath and contamination from that site." Although the authors noted that "for long-term IUD users, the relative risk of pelvic inflammatory disease (PID) was 15.6 percent for those using the Dalkon Shield" they did not think it necessary to attempt to identify and notify women who might still be at risk. They reasoned that "the manufacturer advised physicians to remove the Dalkon Shield even from asymptomatic patients in 1980. By the end of 1983, essentially all of these patients should have cycled through the physician's office and received that recommendation. Therefore, any attempt to identify and recall the remaining Dalkon Shields would certainly be time consuming and impractical and is probably unnecessary."[89]

In September 1984 *Family Planning Perspectives* published a notice that their clinics had been advised to remove Dalkon Shields from all patients who still wore them. They said, "The risk of pelvic infection increases with the length of time the Dalkon Shield is used. Although the device has been off the market since 1975, many thousands of women may still have the device in place."[90] In October 1984 the A. H. Robins Corporation publicly recommended removal of Dalkon Shields from women wearing them. They claimed that "new" information revealed that the risk of IUD use increased the longer a device was worn and announced that the corporation would pay for removals. Two years later, the corporation set a deadline for the filing of Dalkon Shield injury claims. By the deadline, claims had been filed by 306,931 women worldwide.[91] Thousands of claims had already been "cleared" by the corporation and its insurer. An estimated four and a half million women had used the Dalkon Shield; approximately 8 percent of those women filed claims. The actual incidence of injury and death is unknown.

Commercial bias and the faulty design of the Dalkon Shield form only an incomplete explanation for the magnitude of the risk faced by women in this case. Several risk-inducing factors for Dalkon Shield users are relevant to users of all intrauterine devices.

Examining the medical literature on IUDs, I found that authors of articles on IUD performance and safety are often the inventors of the devices they claim to evaluate objectively. The promotion of the Dalkon Shield by Hugh J. Davis and other paid consultants of the A. H. Robins Corporation was not an unusual practice, although that promotion may have been unusually vigorous. No financial or professional interest of medical investigators reporting on IUDs was disclosed in any of the articles I found by inventors of IUDs.

There was little consensus in the medical literature on any point relative to the use of IUDs. As is standard in medical discussion of any controversial product or practice, debate characterized every issue. Subjective considerations, personal values, and biases marked each discussion. Professional assessment of IUD performance generally involved consideration of relative risks and comparison of IUDs to each other, to other methods of contraception, and to pregnancy. The absolute risk of IUD use has never been established; for any given woman, the absolute risk cannot be known.

Medical investigators found that the Dalkon Shield had some structural peculiarities that probably increased the likelihood of infection and other injuries. The courts concluded that the device was defective and that the case was handled negligently by the corporation and its representatives. Some observers believe that the Dalkon Shield was dangerous, but that other IUDs are safe. This study suggests that the risks inherent in the use of all IUDs may have been intensified by the specific design and the particular way in which the Dalkon Shield case was handled. But the medical literature reported problems with *all* intrauterine devices. Those problems included chronic and acute infection, perforations, infertility, complicated pregnancies, injury to and loss of vital body parts and functions, and death.

Despite the injuries reported, some medical investigators continue to assert that intrauterine devices are safe when handled properly and prescribed appropriately. Other investigators claim that the biologic effects of intrauterine devices invite complications. They suggest that the contraceptive effect of an intrauterine device is produced by the same mechanisms and reactions that predispose the user to injury. Disagreement by experts on issues crucial to women's health marked the history of the Dalkon Shield case. Failure to understand that all medical "knowledge" is subject to such debate is itself a source of substantial risk to all consumers of medical products and services.

3   Class, Race, and Country

Experts in the fields of medicine and family planning have consistently maintained that certain populations of women need birth control more desperately than others. Poor women everywhere, and particularly poor women in "developing" countries, are said to have the most pressing need. Occasionally, the health and well-being of individual women and their children has been the focus of professional concern. High maternal and infant mortality rates have been cited to bolster the claim that pregnancy, for some women, is more dangerous than any available method of birth control. Professionals have sometimes justified the mass use of contraceptive products that carry substantial risks on that basis.

More often, professionals cite the health and well-being of large populations—sometimes of all humanity—as their primary concern. They claim that overpopulation causes economic and social problems on a global scale, an assertion supported by traditional demographic theory. Stable population size is said to characterize "preindustrial" societies. Birthrates are high, but so are death rates. With industrialization, death rates drop and birthrates remain high. The consequent explosion of population growth is said to cause a strain on natural and economic resources. According to this theory, further development is impeded, and poverty, hunger, illness, and social unrest originate in this population expansion.

Eugenicists fear that rapid population growth in indigent populations will mean that humanity will be weakened by "inferior genetic stock." Professionals with more pedestrian interests have joined them in their support of drastic measures of population control. Fearing that "overpopulation" among the poor will "breed revolution," prominent members of the family planning community have focused their concern on the preservation of what they refer to as "civilization as we know it."

In 1970, *Life* magazine published an article featuring the philosophy and work of Dr. Paul Ehrlich and Dr. Thomas Eisner, cofounders of the group Zero Population Growth, or ZPG. A campus-based organization initiated at Yale University, ZPG boasted "102 chapters in 30 states" at the time the article was written. The group directed its efforts toward education and political pressure to curb global population growth. The human species, they believed, would otherwise "breed itself literally to extinction."

The author of that article lamented that "a certain cold and dispassionate cast of mind is required in order to regard the birth of human life not as a joyous event but as a proliferation of some deadly malignancy."[1] The author's claim that this was "precisely the view held" by proponents of population control was well substantiated. The year before, Dr. Alan Guttmacher, who for many years was president of the Planned Parenthood Federation of America and chairperson of the International Planned Parenthood Federation, described the population "crisis" in this way: "It strikes me that civilization, as we know it, is less threatened by cancer than by the present epidemic of human beings."[2]

Concern about this "epidemic" dominated popular and professional literature on the subject of birth control in the 1960s and early 1970s. In 1971, the Population Crisis Committee published a collection of essays entitled *Population Research: Mankind's Great Need*. The thirty essays in the collection were written by men with impressive credentials. All known methods of birth control were discussed, with the exception of barrier methods. No mention was made in any essay of women's desire to control their procreative power. An appeal for financial support for contraceptive research was made on the basis of the urgent need to curb the "burgeoning" world population.[3]

In recent years the basic tenets of traditional demographic theory have been challenged. Demographers have found that the relationship of fertility rates to social and economic conditions is complex and culturally specific. According to Betsy Hartmann, the nature of the relationship can be better understood by changing the definition of development: "If one measures development simply in terms of GNP per capita, then one finds that countries with higher per capita income generally have lower birth rates, though there are important exceptions to this rule. . . . If one defines development differently, in terms of the number of people who actually benefit from economic growth, then one discovers that more equitable distribution of resources can lead to lower birth rates, even at relatively low levels of GNP per capita." This analysis reverses the traditional assertion that lower birthrates are necessary to bring about a higher standard of living. According to Hartmann, until "a raised standard of living across the population leads to better overall access to health, education and jobs," many poor families will not be able to afford to have fewer children. Contrary to the expectations of traditionalists, children are often, under specific economic and social conditions, economic assets, contributing more to the family through productive labor than they consume.[4]

At the time that the Dalkon Shield was marketed, the belief that overpopulation was the primary cause of the world's growing economic and social problems prevailed. The idea that the health of individual women using potentially dangerous methods of contraception could justifiably be risked for the good of mankind dominated the literature. In 1970 Garrett Hardin wrote, "As of the moment, the IUD is the greatest hope for the poor countries of the world. Even when it fails to work for ten percent of the women, it is a blessing to the country as a whole. The woman who becomes pregnant in spite of an IUD insertion is unlucky indeed; but a starving country that can prevent ninety percent of the births that aren't wanted is richer thereby and may be able to lift itself out of the trap of poverty." Recommendations for a double standard of medical treatment, depending on socioeconomic circumstances, were rife throughout the medical and population control literature. Hardin claimed that the exclusive use of licensed professionals to "install" IUDs in the United States could be "defended" on the basis that "in the process of inserting an IUD a trained physician may spot some health condition that needs treatment." He believed, however, that "one day's supervised training" would be "adequate to prepare intelligent paramedics to carry out this function" in poor countries. Hardin explained, "Since they are generally short of both doctors and money (and long on babies) poor countries cannot afford the luxury of restricting this practice to M.D.'s."[5]

Intrauterine devices were hailed as "the greatest hope for poor countries" in part because they "cost only a penny or so in wholesale lots." According to Hardin,

> The inserters cost a little bit more but, with intervening sterilization, it can be used over and over. In a rich country like ours, which is well supplied with doctors and in which the time of skilled people is expensive, it is common practice to use packaged, pre-sterilized IUD and inserter only once, throwing away the inserter after use. This "wastefulness" may make the best use of expensive professional time. In poor countries, however, time is more abundant than money, and the inserter can be used repeatedly.[6]

To Dr. Alan Guttmacher, the speed with which IUDs could be inserted made them particularly appropriate for use in poor countries where, in his analysis, professional time was limited. Guttmacher described IUD insertions that he had witnessed in Hong Kong.

> The best IUD manipulator I have ever observed was in Hong Kong. . . . Her record was seventy-five insertions in three hours. I have figured that out, that is one every two minutes and twenty-four seconds. Dr. Wong kept three nurses busy helping her. One was supervising the removal of the panties of the next patient, the second nurse soothed the brow of the patient on the table and the third passed instruments to Dr. Wong. I have never seen such graceful hands, such exquisite economy of finger movement; there wasn't a false motion. I regret that I am not a choreographer, for a ballet of IUD patients with the ballerina making Dr. Wong's finger and hand movements would be a sensation.[7]

The process that Guttmacher described more closely approximated Taylorism and the assembly line than any ballet. What the assembly line produced was a situation of substantial risk for the women receiving IUDs. In the "two minutes and twenty-four seconds" accorded each patient, a thorough examination to determine the woman's physical and anatomical condition would not have been possible, and it is questionable whether sterile precautions could have been rigidly adhered to. If one inserter was used repeatedly in this performance, sterile conditions were certainly compromised.

Potential contamination of the intrauterine environment by bacteria introduced during the insertion process did not worry Guttmacher.

> Contrary to experience of a half century ago, the use of an IUD is not associated with a high incidence of pelvic infection. It appears that bacteria are always introduced into the uterine cavity with the insertion of an IUD, but the cavity has a marvelous capacity to sterilize itself within seventy-two hours and after this time almost always gives a negative culture. If pelvic infection occurs with an IUD in place, it can be treated effectively with antibiotics without removing the device.[8]

The actual incidence of pelvic infection associated with the use of IUDs has been a subject of controversy for many decades. In 1968 the U.S. Food and Drug Administration determined the incidence sufficient to justify a recommendation that sterile precautions be maximized with all IUD insertions.[9] Guttmacher supported the use of "itinerant teams" of family planning workers that would "visit villages to insert IUDs and then not return until months later." If those teams employed the methods Guttmacher witnessed and admired in Hong Kong, women who were put at risk by minimal attention to sterile precautions during the insertion process would have that risk intensified by the absence of medical and follow-up treatment "until months later."

In his book promoting intrauterine devices in general and his Dalkon Shield in particular, Dr. Hugh Davis lamented the "terrifying" population growth "in Asia, Africa and Latin America." With particular reference to India, Davis warned that "young people already born" would soon be "spawning additional millions of progeny." The solution Davis proposed was mass use of birth control, especially intrauterine devices.[10] Davis suggested differential treatment under varying circumstances for women who suffered uterine perforations.

> Rare cases of intestinal obstruction have occurred due to entrapment of a segment of a bowel in an open loop device which has only partially perforated a uterus. For that reason, we have advocated removal of the device as the wisest choice of action. Under conditions of mass use in primitive circumstances, it can be argued that most uterine perforations do not result in

significant morbidity, that the device is relatively inert, and that its presence in an extrauterine location may be ignored with relative safety. Nevertheless, when circumstances permit, removal of the ectopic device is desirable.[11]

Many physicians and population control experts have stressed the importance that women accept methods of birth control that assure maximum effectiveness in preventing pregnancy and require minimum action or motivation on the woman's part. In 1968 the U.S. Food and Drug Administration identified underprivileged women as a population more effectively served with IUDs, because with those devices "the need for recurrent motivation, required in other forms of contraception, is removed."[12]

Professionals also give close attention to acceptance rates and retention or continuation rates in their comparative evaluation of birth control methods and products. In 1970, Clive Wood wrote, "Developing nations [are] areas where the population particularly needs a method of birth control showing a high continuation rate." Furthermore, in Wood's view, "The younger women in any given population are more fertile than the older ones and a primary aim of any national program of birth control must be to provide effective contraception for them specifically." Wood bemoaned what he called the "neighborhood effect" for its influence on continuation rates. He wrote, "The knowledge that one woman had had sufficient difficulty with her device to have it removed may cause some friends, who have themselves had no trouble, to assume that the method must be bad and should be abandoned. This 'neighborhood effect' should not be underestimated, particularly in regions where educational standards are low." Wood prescribed a preventive or cure for the so-called neighborhood effect. For women who could not be persuaded to use or to continue using IUDs, he suggested government intervention in the form of economic sanctions. He wrote, "A government-financed scheme in which it was in the woman's economic interest to have a device inserted and to keep it there (or failing that, to have one re-inserted) might make a great deal of difference to the discontinuation rate in many parts of the world."[13]

Wood was not merely concerned with women who might wish to stop using IUDs because of problems they had experienced or had heard about. He was also concerned that women were free to choose to have their IUDs removed in order to become pregnant.

> The desire for another pregnancy motivates a (fortunately small) number of women to have the IUD removed. I say "fortunately" because the physician is unlikely to persuade such a woman to change her mind, although the consequences of her action for the population as a whole are obvious. . . . Until strong personal disincentives to have more children are introduced by the governments of the world, the physician, faced with such a request, will never have any alternative but to remove the device.[14]

The material consequences of the ideological assertions and recommendations espoused by powerful leaders in the family planning community were manifest in public policy by the time the Dalkon Shield was marketed. Population control programs had become multimillion-dollar enterprises backed by governments, private foundations, and industry. More than four and a half million Dalkon Shields were distributed by private physicians, birth control clinics, and itinerant teams of family planning workers in eighty countries during a period of approximately four years. In many areas incentive programs had been initiated to encourage women to accept and retain IUDs. There were three features that made the Dalkon Shield attractive for use in those programs: it was inexpensive; it was designed to make expulsion (and removal) difficult; and it was made in a size that allegedly made it suitable for young women who had never been pregnant.

The targeting of particular women by population control programs created significant risks for those who turned to those programs for help in controlling their procreative power. A woman's choice of contraceptive method was limited by what was made available to her and by what she could afford. Her choice might be influenced by the incentives attached to products that professionals wished her to choose. Some programs did not offer the illusion of choice. A woman's health would be influenced by the sterile or septic conditions under which she was treated by clinic personnel. Her chances of survival in case of infection or other injury would be influenced by her proximity to medical facilities adequate to treat her condition and by the time, expertise, availability, and willingness of personnel to perform those services for her.

These conditions make class, race, and country important in any assessment of risks faced by women who use contraceptive products. The targeting of poor women for differential treatment by professionals implies that a gap must exist between the experiences of women of different social circumstances. If there is a gap, a correspondence might also exist between relative class, race, and national status and the intensity of risk and injury a given woman is expected to suffer.

The interviews I conducted for this project yielded a more complex picture. All the women were residents of the United States; a majority were white; half would be considered comfortably middle class or upper class by any standard of sociological measurement. Many sources of risk identified in this sample were class specific. There were differences in the nature of some of the risks these women faced, in the timing of exposure to risks, and in their opportunities to escape or modify some of the consequences of injury once it occurred. But none of these women escaped exposure to risks. The more privileged women were exposed to some sources of risk particular to women of their own class and deeply rooted in their class privilege.

Four of the most economically and socially advantaged women in this study dominated their narratives with self-conscious (and class-conscious) assertions of the "kind of person" each believed herself to be. These women saw themselves as educated, aware, and informed consumers. They chose the best physicians, consulted them on a regular basis, and worked actively with them to make what they believed were sound personal and medical decisions. These women valued active participation in their own health care and believed that their health depended on this kind of responsible behavior. Their concepts of themselves as women in control of their destinies caused them some specific problems.

Anna was a twenty-one-year-old single college student when she received her Dalkon Shield in 1971. After suffering silent pelvic inflammatory disease, Anna learned to her surprise that she had become infertile. Her oviducts had become blocked with scar tissue from the infection.

Surgery to repair her oviducts was unsuccessful, and it was only after several attempts at in vitro fertilization that Anna was finally able to conceive the child she desperately wanted to bear. When I met Anna in 1986, she was a college professor who had married and was the mother of an infant conceived in vitro.

Anna said that she chose a Dalkon Shield because it was presented to her as the "avant-garde IUD." As a single woman, Anna trusted those physicians who were willing to help her to get birth control against her parents' wishes. She said she was "the type of person at the time who was not ambivalent about not wanting children." She was a "great believer in birth control . . . one of those emancipated women." When a health care provider at a European clinic advised Anna to have her Dalkon Shield removed immediately if she ever wanted to have children, Anna ignored her, thinking "this poor woman, she doesn't know anything about the miracles of American birth control."

In time Anna deeply regretted her "haughty" attitude. She said that she had been "the perfect dupe." What Anna thought she knew about the Dalkon Shield had been false and misleading. She, like millions of other women and many of the health care providers who served them, initially believed that the Dalkon Shield was a superior IUD, a revolutionary new device that—as one woman expressed it—"was going to solve all our problems." It is impossible to know how extensively Anna had already been injured when she was advised to have her Dalkon Shield removed. The delay brought about by what Anna "knew" about the "miracles of American birth control" and by her disrespect for the clinic worker's opinion may have cost Anna her fertility. It could have cost her her life.

As a woman deeply invested in her sense of herself as a person who could direct her own destiny, Anna was tormented with guilt when she learned that she could not get pregnant because she had been injured by her Dalkon Shield. Anna said, "At the time that I first found out about my infertility I became so—unbelievably totally—hysterical that I was going through my diaries and I was quizzing everyone—my old boyfriend, my mother, just everyone. I was trying to relive this and get it all straight in my mind if I was guilty, because I just felt so tormented by this."

Anna blamed herself for having been "such a rebel" that she failed to go to "better doctors." She blamed her parents for having "put up an enormous stink about adolescent sexuality." She blamed her mother in particular for not "involving herself more" in Anna's health care and for not taking her to "a decent doctor." Anna expressed some ambivalence about the culpability of her health care providers. She said she thought her "story could have happened with the finest doctors" but she also said, "Possibly if I'd been going to a better doctor they would have removed it sooner."

Anna's reasoning was paradoxical. The health care providers she had chosen had not failed to warn her that her Dalkon Shield should be removed; she had failed to heed their warning. If a physician Anna had respected had given her the same warning, she might have allowed that physician to remove the device. In that case, the device would have been removed sooner not because the physician was objectively superior but because Anna considered that physician a "better doctor." By attempting to allay her guilt for the delay by blaming it on inferior health care providers, Anna forced herself into a position of guilt by virtue of her having chosen those providers. While her reasoning offered her no tenable defense against her own feelings of guilt, it did reassure her that the norms of her social class—against which she had temporarily and regrettably rebelled—were defensible.

The behavioral imperatives of Anna's social class demanded that she plan every aspect of her life and direct those plans to fruition, so she experienced her infertility as an affront to her self-esteem. Only through planning an alternate route to parenthood could Anna save herself from despair. Guilt, torment, and depression were potentially lethal. Anna said that she "saw the limits of what [she] could bear" as she waited through the period of uncertainty before she finally became pregnant. She did not know "what would have happened" if she "had been tested more than that." She felt that if she could not carry out her plan to give birth to a child "it would have been rational to commit suicide."

Donna was another affluent woman who suffered self-recriminations for her agency in having used the Dalkon Shield. Donna suffered severe injuries from her use of that device. She had pelvic inflammatory disease that left extensive scarring in her oviducts, suffered a ruptured ectopic pregnancy that required two episodes of major abdominal surgery in a period of three weeks, and later had a miscarriage that she believed might have been related to her injuries. Donna thought about suing the A. H. Robins Corporation but hesitated to do so, struggling with her ambivalence about who or what was responsible for her injuries.

Donna had one "successful" pregnancy after using the Dalkon Shield and before the ectopic pregnancy; she had a second "successful" pregnancy later, after undergoing reconstructive surgery to repair her oviducts. She considered her children evidence of her personal success at overcoming her injuries through wise medical choices. She had a great deal of difficulty acknowledging that she had ever been less than successful at protecting herself by keeping well informed. When she did recognize that she had been injured because she had been misled by false information, her view of herself as a person in control of her life was challenged. Not to acknowledge that she had been misled would have put her in the position of assuming full responsibility for her injuries because she chose the Dalkon Shield. Her difficulty in resolving that conflict was apparent throughout her interview.

Donna stressed that she heeded information when making birth control decisions. She had originally used the pill, she said, "because I definitely didn't want to get pregnant and it was known to be the absolute safest *way* to guard against pregnancy, so I went on the pill and nobody was talking about side effects then." Donna stopped taking the pill for a while, and when she needed birth control again she said that she "didn't want to go back on the pill because by that point side effects were being talked about and by then the commonly known method that was supposed to be the safest to prevent pregnancy without the side effects of the *pill* was the IUD, and the Dalkon Shield was known (I remember) for being good for women who'd never had babies, who've never been pregnant with smaller uteruses or something, they were supposed to give less trouble and be rejected by your body less."

When Donna purchased her Dalkon Shield in 1971, all the literature available on the device carried the information she remembered. It was printed in medical journals, often in articles authored or coauthored by Dr. Hugh J. Davis; it was in the promotional literature given to physicians and patients; and it was also included in the feminist health book *Our Bodies, Ourselves.* I asked Donna if she remembered where she might have heard the information, and she responded, "I really don't remember. It just seemed to be—maybe it was in all the literature about the Dalkon Shield, you know, I'm the kind of *person* who keeps well informed about these things and the current methods, and, and, I just remember being, I mean that's what everyone knew around me."

Donna had difficulty reconciling her sense of herself as well informed and responsible for her own actions with her memory of the actual process by which she came to use the Dalkon Shield. She explained that the doctor she consulted was a private physician. Like Anna, Donna apparently felt that to choose a private physician was more responsible than to attend a public clinic. Donna was uncertain, however, whether she wanted to say that it was she or her physician who was responsible for the decision that she would use the Dalkon Shield. She alternated the subject pronouns "I" and "he," saying, "I went to a doctor—a private physician—and he—I asked for an IUD—and he—actually I—I mean he did say that, you know, the Dalkon Shield would be the best for somebody who never had a baby so that's what I got."

Donna was asked if she saw a physician during the two years that she had the Dalkon Shield and her response was, "I imagine I did because I tend to 'do what you're supposed to do' and go to the doctor every year so I must have at least once." By stressing that she was the kind of person who consistently acted responsibly on behalf of her own health, Donna implied that she questioned her own culpability for having used the Dalkon Shield. She tried to resolve that issue by presenting evidence that she had done everything that she was supposed to do to protect herself.

Donna presented herself as an authority on the issues discussed in her interview. She responded defensively several times when asked to clarify her remarks. At one point she presented "figures" that she had learned from her physician. In answer to the question, "Did the doctor ever indicate to you why you had an ectopic pregnancy?" Donna said:

> Well, you know he definitely said that there was scar tissue when he first went in and that it could have been—it was probably definitely due to that bad infection that I had—he did say that it could have been due to the Dalkon Shield but—you know—he said that you never know for sure about these things. He *did* say that in his experience the *rate* of tubal pregnancies in the New York area which is one area which experiences a lot of women using birth control methods had gone from an average of one in *three* hundred to one in seventy in the ten years that he had been practicing.

I asked Donna, "Was that among all women . . . ?" and she interrupted with the retort, "It was in *general,* I don't know, the *average.* I don't know what studies he was basing it on, but he did use those figures—one in three hundred and one in seventy—it more than tripled." Donna moved quickly from her remark that the physician said her injuries were "probably definitely" due to the infection she contracted when she had the Dalkon Shield to her discussion of the physician's general experience with an increase in tubal pregnancies. By citing the "figures," Donna shed some doubt on the Dalkon Shield's responsibility for causing her injuries. It was among women in "an area which experiences a lot of people using birth control"—not specifically among women who used the Dalkon Shield—that ectopic pregnancies had increased. Donna's knowledge of those figures buttressed her claim that she was "the kind of person who keeps well informed about these things." In addition, her comments affirmed her respect for her physician's authority on such matters, and offered assurance that she chose a knowledgeable physician who shared information with her.

Both Donna and Anna made it clear at the beginning of their interviews that they were not ambivalent about the prospect of becoming pregnant. Anna said that she was "not ambivalent about not wanting children" and Donna said she "definitely didn't want to get pregnant."

Both women felt that an unambiguous desire to use birth control effectively was an important part of being the type of person each was supposed to be. This was one source of risk for these women, because it meant that they sought contraceptive effectiveness over contraceptive safety. Donna was among several women I interviewed who used the word *safety* in reference to the method's ability to prevent pregnancy—as opposed to its physical effect upon the body.

Mary was another woman who emphasized the importance of working closely with one's own private physicians and keeping informed and educated on matters relevant to one's health. Mary had open-heart surgery before she used the Dalkon Shield. Her choice of contraceptive method was limited by her heart condition, and her need for an effective method of contraception was urgent. She could not risk pregnancy, and she could not risk using oral contraceptives. The anesthesia and surgery necessary for a tubal ligation would have been dangerous. An IUD seemed to be an ideal choice for her.

Mary had to have her Dalkon Shield removed after it "went bad" and caused her a severe pelvic infection that required hospitalization and almost resulted in hysterectomy. Mary described the sudden onset of her pelvic infection. She said, "I didn't feel terribly bad, I just didn't feel *right*. . . . I started with a sharp pain that got progressively worse. I was surprised at how fast I went bad; I don't think I ever had anything that went bad so fast—I mean infections or sickness, or what have you, that bad—that fast. That really shocked me—the time element."

Despite the obvious risks inherent in that "time element," Mary said:

> I think they should still manufacture the IUD. I think that people—are put in such a fix—with birth control methods—that there are certain—you can elect to take a risk. As long as it's a very clear risk—and they're a little more careful about whom they put them in. . . . I mean—if I was—educated and aware enough to attempt to use the pill and have a problem and go off it, and having the IUD and have a problem, you know—there are risks in everything, and where the risk of pregnancy is greater than with the IUD—who's in a position to make that judgment? It's like the abortion issue, who's in a position to make that judgment but you yourself?

Mary's analysis was inconsistent with her own experience. She had suffered what she called "ministrokes" while using the pill; she had suffered pelvic inflammatory disease while using the Dalkon Shield. Either of these conditions could have been fatal. Mary was fortunate to have had time to stop taking the pill, and she was fortunate that her Dalkon Shield could be removed before more extensive injuries occurred. In both cases Mary stopped using the method because she became suddenly and critically ill, not because she was "educated and aware." Furthermore, while pregnancy may or may not have been more dangerous for her than these methods of contraception proved to be, pregnancy was not her only alternative to the use of these methods. Barrier methods—rejected by Mary for reasons unrelated to her health—could have provided contraceptive protection equal to or greater than that provided by the pill or the IUD.

Confidence in the value of her information and education as insurance against injury marked the testimony of a fourth woman. Ursula never used the Dalkon Shield; she used a series of four Copper 7 devices. She gave contradictory testimony about her experiences. First, she explained that her fourth Copper 7 had been removed because it had caused an inflammation in her uterus; then she claimed that she had never had a problem with that method of contraception. Confronted with the apparent contradiction, Ursula explained that an inflammation was not the same thing as an infection.

Ursula believed she was the kind of person who could safely use an IUD. She said, "I think that for *me,* who has a single sexual partner, and particularly now, when I don't want to have other kids, I don't have to worry about—the scarring that might take place." Ursula's comment reflected her acceptance of four popular misconceptions: (1) that the number of a woman's sexual partners will determine her exposure to infection; (2) that IUD-related infection is usually sexually transmitted; (3) that the only serious complication associated with the use of IUDs is infection; and (4) that infertility is the only serious consequence of IUD injury. Ursula also believed that the problems associated with the Dalkon

Shield resulted from its unique properties and did not apply to other IUDs.

There are several problems with Ursula's analysis. A woman's own sexual practices do not absolutely determine her risk of exposure to sexually transmitted infection. A monogamous woman whose sexual partner is not monogamous is exposed to the same chain of sexual contacts as her partner. And while most experts claim that a woman having more than one sexual partner increases her risk of infection, some studies have shown an inverse relationship. One study found that among short-term IUD users, women who reported having more than one sexual partner were less likely to be hospitalized for a first incidence of pelvic inflammatory disease than women who reported having only one sexual partner. They also found that women having sexual intercourse more than five times a week were less likely to be hospitalized for a first incidence of this kind of infection than were women with less frequent sexual contact.[15] While these results are controversial, they indicate that assumption of a causal relationship between sexual habits and infection is problematic.

Many studies have shown that women wearing intrauterine devices are more likely to become ill with pelvic inflammatory disease than are women without them. Estimates vary, but most experts now concur that the risk for users is five to nine times greater than for nonusers. Several infections are included under the rubric "pelvic inflammatory disease." Some are sexually transmitted; others can be transmitted through the bloodstream from other parts of the woman's own body. Infectious organisms may ascend from the lower genital tract to invade the uterus, oviducts, and pelvic area. Some of these organisms are harmless to the vagina but potentially lethal once they cross the cervix. Many IUD-related infections result from bacteria introduced as the device is inserted. Others begin when an IUD perforates the bowel, bladder, or appendix. It is therefore possible for a woman who uses an IUD to become infected without ever having sexual contact.[16]

In the absence of an IUD, intrauterine infection is said to be "extremely rare." While some experts claim that this is due to the uterus' ability to sterilize itself, others claim that all healthy, intact tissue is resistant to infection.[17] Problems occur once an IUD is introduced because "an IUD is capable of inducing changes that can lead to inflammatory and infectious diseases, separately or together."[18] As we have seen, many researchers believe that IUDs work to prevent pregnancy by setting up an inflammatory reaction. Julian Elias explained:

> It is now generally accepted that the main contraceptive action of the IUD is the production of a sterile inflammatory reaction in the uterus. This occurs as a result of a foreign body being present in the cavity. The breakdown products of these inflammatory cells are toxic to sperm and blastocysts. The smaller the device, the less the inflammatory reaction produced, which would explain the higher pregnancy rate with smaller devices. The addition of copper to a small device increases the inflammatory reaction.[19]

Dr. Waldemar Schmidt described the "surface coating" that normally forms "not only on the IUD but on the tail as well." He wrote, "The organic surface-coat is composed of mucoid and cellular elements. The cellular elements have been shown by electron microscopy to consist of an inflammatory response, the cellular composition of which changes over time. . . . Its significance is revealed by the pathogenic bacterial flora that come to inhabit this new ecological niche."[20]

Ursula stated that she believed that inflammation and infection were two different conditions. Clive Wood commented in 1971,

> Investigators have failed to make a clear distinction between infection and inflammation. Medical dictionaries define the former as a condition set up by the presence of pathogenic organisms. . . . The reaction of tissue to an inert foreign body is in many ways similar to its reaction to a pathogen, and many pathologists would agree that to distinguish an infected tissue from one undergoing a sterile foreign body response, on histological evidence alone, is an extremely difficult task. This is precisely the reason why attention has been drawn to the criteria that various investigators have employed when diagnosing endometritis in patients showing no clinical symptoms of such a complaint.[21]

The problem with this analysis is that it seeks to distinguish inflammation from infection without identifying the relationship that appears to exist between the two processes, as shown by Dr. Schmidt's explanation that once an allegedly "sterile" inflammatory response occurs, "pathogenic bacterial flora . . . come to inhabit this new ecological niche."

A group of physicians discussed this relationship with reference to the body's immune response. They wrote, "Once colonization has taken place, host factors (immune responses) may play an all-important role in containing the infectious process. . . . Immunosuppressive and debilitating conditions and trauma are predisposing factors." It has been postulated that a relationship encouraging colonization of bacteria exists between a foreign body reaction and immune responses. In 1976 Drs. Michael Colin and Gerald Weissman described this relationship. They wrote, "Within the uterus, local defense mechanisms are important in preventing infection. The intrauterine device, a foreign body, invokes a cell-mediated, immune response in the adjacent endometrium; macrophages migrate and adhere to that device."[22] The macrophages, the authors explained, secrete a substance known as "prostaglandin E_1."

> Since prostaglandin E_1 may delay . . . a process necessary for bacterial killing, the intercellular persistence of micro-organisms might be favored by release of prostaglandin E_1, from macrophages adherent to the device. Conceivably, within the intrauterine milieu, this altered inflammatory response in the presence of an intrauterine device may [contribute] to the dissemination of [a] patient's localized infection. Furthermore, the mechanisms may help account for the increased frequency of pelvic inflammatory disease in wearers of such devices.[23]

According to this analysis, the "sterile" inflammatory foreign body reaction within the uterus suppresses the immune responses and at the same time attracts colonies of pathogenic bacteria. This process alters the environment in which the IUD rests, making disease likely to flourish in the presence of infectious bacteria. A number of microorganisms have been isolated in cases of pelvic inflammatory disease in women using IUDs, including streptococcus pneumoniae, E-coli, B-streptococcus, and actinomyces.[24] Each of these infections is capable of invading the uterine and pelvic areas through means other than sexual contact.

In recent years case reports of actinomycosis have dominated the literature on pelvic inflammatory disease. According to Dr. Waldemar

Schmidt, "Fatal cases of actinomycetales infection associated with intra-uterine foreign bodies were reported in 1928 . . . and in 1930. . . . The full significance of such complications, however, [was] not fully appreciated until the [last] quarter of the 20th century." Actinomycosis has been described as "one of the most problematic IUD-related infections." Women infected with actinomycosis tend to appear asymptomatic; the disease is difficult to diagnose until it is well advanced. Actinomyces normally inhabit dental cavities and are found in persons with gingivitis, periodontitis, infected root canals, and dental calculus. They have also been found in wound infections, sinus infections, and in particular forms of gall bladder and thyroid disease. It has been postulated that these organisms can be transmitted through the bloodstream from other infected parts of a woman's own body, or from orogenital contact with an infected partner. Some researchers believe that "a defective local antibody response might also be a contributing factor for the development of actinomycosis."[25]

The long-term consequences of a single episode of pelvic infection can be dramatic. According to Theodore Nagel, "The risk of tubal occlusion after a single episode of infection is 12.9%. For gonococcal pelvic infection the risk is 6.1% and for non-gonococcal it is 17.3%." Stadel and Schlesselman studied "a wide range of United States hospitals" and found that "about 8% of women hospitalized with a first episode of pelvic inflammatory disease have extensive disease (defined as pelvic inflammatory disease treated by hysterectomy or bilateral adnexal surgery, with pelvic inflammatory disease as the only gynecologic discharge diagnosis)."[26]

It is difficult to judge the severity of disease by the treatment received, particularly when that treatment is hysterectomy. Regardless of the severity of disease, however, the risk that a hysterectomy or ovariectomy will be performed if infection occurs is faced by every woman who uses an IUD. The likelihood that these operations will be performed depends on the physician's attitudes, the woman's age, the number of her children, her race, and her social class. These operations have their own risks. The study of long-term effects of hysterectomy and ovariectomy has been grossly neglected by medical research, but hysterectomy and ovariectomy are known to influence the circulatory, endocrine, and nervous systems, as well as libido and sexual response.[27]

In 1973 Dr. Simon Henderson published a case report that sparked interest within the medical community about the link between actinomycosis and intrauterine devices. A thirty-eight-year-old woman had been admitted to the hospital with lower abdominal pain, nausea, and "a heavy yellow discharge." Physicians initially thought that she had endometriosis. Her general physical condition was found to be unremarkable except that she had teeth that were very "carious and accompanied by severe gingivitis." Abdominal surgery revealed that:

> A tubo-ovarian mass ∴ . . was plastered to the right pelvic sidewall. The terminal ileum and numerous loops of bowel were adherent to the superior and posterior aspects of the mass. . . . The uterus was normal in appearance except for bilateral tubo adhesions. The left tube was thickened and elongated so that the fimbrial end was firmly attached to the perirectal . . . mass deep in the left side of the pelvis. . . . The left ovary . . . was adherent to the lateral part of the uterus.

As a result of these findings "a total abdominal hysterectomy was performed with considerable difficulty in removing the right adnexal mass because of its adherent nature and the proximity of the ureter, which had to be carefully identified and dissected free."[28] This woman had used a Majzlin Spring intrauterine device.

Many women who used the Dalkon Shield became infected with actinomycosis and other infections, which resulted in injuries like those described by Henderson. There has been considerable controversy over whether such cases were more common among Dalkon Shield users than among users of other intrauterine devices. R. Snowden and B. Pearson studied reports of infection in the United Kingdom from 1971 to 1978. They compared the reports associated with the Dalkon Shield, the Gravigard (Copper 7), and two sizes of the Lippes Loop. They found that "there was no significant difference between the four devices when compared to each other over the same period of time." The Centers for Disease Control in Atlanta conducted a study of maternal deaths in the

United States between 1972 and 1974. Of the seventeen IUD-related deaths reported during that period, thirteen were of women who had been using the Dalkon Shield. As late as 1983 researchers were still debating this issue. One comparative study found that "the risk was highest for users of the Dalkon Shield, lowest for users of the copper-containing devices, and intermediate for users of other IUDs, principally the Lippes Loop."[29]

One problem with making these comparisons is that it obscures the important similarities between the Dalkon Shield and other IUDs. The debate addresses the question of relative statistical risks. Women who use other brands of intrauterine devices face absolute—not relative—risks. Another problem with these comparisons was addressed by Schmidt: "Because . . . the tail was so clearly different from the other monofilament IUD strings, the Dalkon Shield infections fell, perhaps by default, into a specific category. This left intact the usual 'gonorrheal type'—PID—syndrome concept as an explanation for modern IUD-related infections." Schmidt believed that the wicking effect of the Dalkon Shield string was partly responsible for some of the problems. He also believed that the surface alterations of the IUD and the string by foreign body reactions may have intensified problems related to the string. And yet another problem may have been created by the large surface area of the Dalkon Shield. The device was designed to maximize contraceptive effect by maximizing surface area; this increased the size of the ecological niche favorable to bacterial colonization. In addition, copper was added to the device, and copper is believed to increase both contraceptive effect and inflammatory reaction.[30]

Many researchers concur that the type of intrauterine device is less important in predicting the likelihood of infection than the duration of use. Stadel and Schlesselman found that duration of use was also related to extent of infection. They wrote, "An IUD that is in place for many years will undergo changes (e.g., harboring of actinomyces) that tend to increase the risk that pelvic inflammatory disease, if it occurs, will be extensive." This problem has led many experts to recommend that IUDs be changed every two years. While this may decrease the colonization of bacteria on each device, it presents another problem, since each time an intrauterine device is removed and another is inserted, there is a risk of bacterial invasion of the uterus. Because many researchers believe that the incidence of infection is highest in the months immediately following insertion, some recommend that IUDs be left alone unless trouble is detected.[31]

Impaired fertility is one serious consequence of IUD injury. There are many others. Injuries documented in the medical literature include: tubal and ovarian pregnancy; spontaneous abortion; septic abortion; fungal infection of the fetus; fetal meningitis; septicemia; bacterial endocarditis; rectouterine fistula; perforation of the uterus; perforation of the bowel; perforation of the bladder; bowel obstruction; urethral obstruction; appendicitis; cervical neoplasia; peritonitis; tubo-ovarian abscess; and pelvic abscess. This is a partial list. All of these injuries can be fatal; many carry the risk of impairment or loss of essential body functions. Many require surgical procedures that entail added risks.[32]

Women of every social description have been injured by intrauterine devices, and all brands of intrauterine devices have caused injuries. The occurrence of injuries is usually determined by factors beyond a woman's control. Neither education nor information is a reliable safeguard against injury. Pregnancy is a potentially lethal complication of IUD use. The failure rate of IUDs averages approximately 3 percent. Because any pregnancy occurring with an IUD is dangerous, physicians usually recommend termination even when the pregnancy is intrauterine and appears normal. When a pregnancy occurs with an IUD in place, the risk that the pregnancy is ectopic is increased.[33]

Impairment of the function of the oviducts is believed to be responsible for the increased risk of ectopic pregnancy. Impairment may occur from infection or from a "sterile" inflammatory reaction similar to that which takes place within the uterus. The oviducts are normally lined with ciliated cells that control the rate of passage of ova, sperm, and blastocysts. With IUD use, the number and motility of ciliated cells are reduced dramatically.[34] Even in normal pregnancy, fertilization takes place in the oviducts. With the impairment of ciliated cells, the zygote can become lodged in the oviduct. The cells multiply, the organisms die, and the oviduct eventually ruptures and bleeds into the pelvic cavity. Surgery is the only treatment for ectopic pregnancy; if it is delayed too long, the woman dies. Because ectopic pregnancies are difficult for physicians to diagnose, the mortality rate is high.

One case report of a woman who became pregnant while using an IUD illustrates the magnitude of risk—informed or otherwise—inherent in the use of IUDs. A thirty-two-year-old woman was admitted to the hospital to have her IUD-related pregnancy terminated. Before the operation she complained of "severe one-sided pelvic pain." According to the physician reporting her case, "The attendant nurse is said to have ascribed this to 'nerves.' After the operation the woman collapsed with severe chest and abdominal pain." The woman was tested for pulmonary embolism, and none was found. After being returned to the general ward the woman "lapsed into a coma." A laparotomy was performed six days after she had been admitted to the hospital. The physicians expected to find a ruptured appendix; they found instead a ruptured ectopic pregnancy. When the case report was published, this woman was "severely brain damaged, practically blind, and quite incapable of caring for her three young children."[35]

The most important limitation of the information women use to make decisions about contraceptive methods is that it is incomplete. The information women receive is influenced by the biases and prejudices of the professionals who provide that information. In the case of the Dalkon Shield, much of that information was tainted by the financial and professional interests of its originator, Dr. Hugh J. Davis, and its manufacturer, the A. H. Robins Corporation. But with all intrauterine devices, the information that has long dominated the popular and professional literature has been influenced by the prolific writings of population control enthusiasts. One physician wrote in protest of that bias in 1970:

> Assessment of the suitability of a contraceptive measure is more dependent on the viewpoint of the assessor than is evaluation of a therapeutic agent employed in the treatment of disease. This is particularly the case with intrauterine devices. Differences of opinion as to the acceptability of the method

exist between physicians whose objective is the provision of family planning advice to the individual patient and those whose primary concern is large-scale population control. It is perhaps unfortunate that the literary output of the latter group of workers greatly exceeds that of the former.[36]

A consideration of the attitudes of physicians toward the health education of their patients gives some insight into the limitations of "informed consent" and the taking of "informed risks." In 1980 Diane Scully conducted interviews with residents in obstetrics and gynecology.

> Every resident indicated a preference for educated rather than uneducated women. However, "educated," as the residents used it, did not mean women who possessed the power of reasoning and judgment or the ability to make knowledgeable decisions. Rather, the term as they used it described middle-class women with middle-class values; that is, those who placed a high premium on good health and who had been taught to respect and submit to the authority of experts. Poor people, the residents believed, lacked middle-class values, were casual about health matters, failed to respond to medical authority, and did not exhibit appropriate deference to physicians. . . . The residents preferred "happy," obedient, respectful and thankful clients.[37]

There was no evidence in my interviews with women to support the assumption that women of one social class place a higher "premium on good health" than women of any other class, but there was ample evidence to suggest that even the most highly educated women were ignorant of female anatomy and physiology and were unaware of the parameters of debate regarding the safety of their contraceptive methods. Anna had her Dalkon Shield removed after several months of suffering with "vaginitis." She said, "The fact that I had become infertile absolutely never crossed my mind. No one ever breathed a word. I do think he felt my tubes and said, 'I think your tubes are O.K.' It wasn't said in such a way that I even knew I had tubes, frankly." Later, when Anna had difficulty conceiving, she consulted another physician. Anna recalled, "The first test the doctor did was a hysterosalpingogram. The guy said to me, how did he put it—he said, "Your right tube is dilated and your left tube is not completely normal." I said, 'What? What's a tube?' I had no idea how this whole business worked."

Most of the information the women did have tended to come from sources that favored efficacy at the expense of safety. Women who, like Anna, did not know that they "even had tubes" could not be said to have been well informed about what they were risking when they used IUDs. While the more affluent women did not see themselves as the type of person who would willingly "submit to the authority of experts," they did express a remarkable respect for that authority and tended to adopt it as their own. Less socially privileged women were more skeptical. For them, material constraints were more likely to influence choices than were ideological positions based on respect for medical authority and knowledge.

Nina was a woman who described herself as "very poor." In 1975 she went to a birth control clinic where she was given an IUD. By that time the Dalkon Shield had been withdrawn from the domestic market. It was not illegal, however, for providers to continue to insert Dalkon Shields that they still had in stock. Nina was not aware at the time that the IUD she was given was a Dalkon Shield. She explained:

> I was living with a man—that—I had a child with and—we didn't have much *money*, we were very poor, and I went to a hospital clinic at that time and that's what they gave me for birth control. I asked them for an IUD. They didn't tell me anything about it; I didn't even find out what I had until later when I had it removed. I was hemorrhaging a lot, and I went back and had it removed. And then the doctor who removed it told me what it was and he said he was very surprised that they had used that because it was not recommended any more at all.

Nina had an opinion about why she had been given a Dalkon Shield when they were "not recommended any more at all." She said, "I don't know why they would do something like that when they know that it's wrong, that it's unhealthy. I don't know how a health professional can do something like that with their conscience. Probably because it was a clinic and the doctor got a low price, maybe the manufacturer was trying to get rid of them."

Nina emphasized that she went to the clinic out of economic need. She first went there to give birth. She said:

I think it was the only clinic in the area from what I knew, because I had come from another state where there was free health care for women, and not at this place, and I had to come back and find my doctor wouldn't take me when I had my first child because I had no hospitalization and no money, and I asked the nurse who taught me Lamaze where I could go and she said the hospital was the only one that had a clinic. It was a dollar a visit, for the doctor's care—and then when I went to have the baby there, on the first day after I had the baby, from the business office they came up and said, "You owe nine hundred dollars to have your baby here, and we want the money before you go home." And he was unemployed at the time that I had the baby, we had no insurance and they kept harassing me about it—and it was a *clinic*.

A change in her economic circumstances led Nina to stop using the clinic after she got her Dalkon Shield. She explained, "I didn't go there after that, I mean, not because of that but my husband had come into his own professionally, since he got a job, so I didn't have to; I guess I wouldn't have been eligible to go there at the time. I think that they use poor people as guinea pigs anyway." Nina believed that it was useless for her to attempt to take legal action against the physician who gave her the Dalkon Shield after it was known to be dangerous. She explained, "It was all clinic, and you really—if you didn't know the doctor personally, you don't really know who you had. It was like a production—it cost a dollar to put it in, and that was it."

Lack of money was just one of the material constraints that influenced working-class and poor women. For both Natalie and Nancy, work-related considerations delayed their getting treatment once problems developed. Natalie, who never knew what brand of IUD had been sold to her at the birth control clinic, told the following story:

I experienced a lot of pain the night I got it. They gave me pain pills—I think codeine—and they told me to take that. And I think they gave me something else—I don't know if it was antibiotics, to combat infection—but I know I had two forms of pills. I couldn't walk home from the clinic, so I took a cab home. I was in a lot of pain, and I was bleeding a lot. But the thing is, I thought it was normal. I mean the nurse that gave the presentation told me that I would experience some cramps, that I would bleed some more.

The first thing I noticed were the cramps and the heavy bleeding. That went on until I had it removed. That didn't stop. It did not end. Every month I had the same thing. But then, the next thing I noticed was that—I worked in a supermarket—and the counters are made of aluminum or something. And they're always very cold. When I was tired, I would lean over the counter. That was just a habit that I had. I would lean over the counter. And then—I think immediately after I got the IUD, I started to experience that whenever I would lean over the counter, the coldness would creep inside me. I would feel the coldness inside. I don't think it was my imagination, because I did not think the IUD was harmful, and I was not connecting it to the IUD—at first.

What happened was, I started getting abdominal pains. Whenever I wore pants that were tight, I would get really severe pain, that I would bend over in pain. And a lot of times it would happen in public, and I would have to like— play it off—and hold in all the pain, and not show people what I was going through. And it happened a lot of times at work, because then whenever I would lean over the counter, it would eventually turn not only to coldness, but I would get pain. And then I became afraid to lean over the counter.

The pain got so bad, I finally went to the hospital. I got the day off from school and from work, and for me to do that, it had to be very bad. I went to the hospital and they immediately took off the IUD. Immediately. The doctor didn't tell me specifically what I had, he just said, "Well, you have this really bad infection, and I have to get this out of you."

Nancy's economic and family circumstances caused her to have to change physicians several times during the year that she had complications from her Dalkon Shield. She was at work when her illness finally became acute.

My husband and I moved—for our family's welfare we moved to wherever he was working, at the time—so I moved that year [1973], soon after I had the IUD inserted. The first infection that I developed was during the fall of that year. I had excruciating pain in my lower abdomen, and felt it was female problems. So I was recommended to see a doctor there, and I visited him, and he said that I had a pelvic infection. That was the time that I found out I had a Dalkon Shield IUD. He recommended that I have it removed because, he said, "This thing could perforate your uterus." But—due to the closeness of my other two children, not being able to accept the pill, I really thought that I had no choice. But this was my first experience with an infection, and hopefully with antibiotics it would clear up, and I would not have any more problems. So, with the antibiotics it did clear up, and I did have no problems for a few months. But it would repeat itself. There was another time during that winter that I had the infection and I was going to my mother's, so I went back to the doctor who inserted it to have him treat me. He gave me antibiotics, and again the infection subsided without difficulty.

This happened three times. In 1974, I had excruciating pain again. But this time it was much, much worse. I started my period that month with a heavy flow, and the flow just never stopped, it just continued. And the pain got worse and worse and worse. I had to work the 3 to 11 shift at the nursing home I was working in ... I told my supervisor of the situation, and she recommended a gynecologist who was directly across the street, and at the dinner hour I called him and he said to come right in, and he immediately removed it. Now, the doctor stated that it was just an irritation, due to the IUD, and that I would experience some cramping, and some flow because of the removal of this. I went back to work that night, and due to lack of staff I had to stay. I was *stuck*. And—through the course of the evening I was just—I mean I had clots the size of—I mean, huge, unbelievable, I did not realize I could pass so much blood and remain—conscious. So, I finished the shift and went home, and fortunately I had the weekend off. I did not get any better. The pain got—increasingly worse. I called the doctor. He told me to take Bufferin. I said, "I have gone through every old medicine in the house." I said that I even had Tylenol with codeine, which just took the edge off this pain. I said, "It's just unbearable!" He said, "Well, we wouldn't suggest anything else."

So, by Sunday night, I believe, I finally had to admit myself to the hospital, because I just could not stand it any longer. I went to the emergency room. They put me in a separate cubicle because by that time I had developed a fever. And they admitted me. I had a *severe* pelvic infection.

Despite the material conditions that separate women from each other, there were similar ideological and material conditions influencing all the women interviewed who used IUDs. For women to "accept" and to "retain" IUDs, it was often necessary for them to endure months of pain and heavy bleeding. Two strategies emerged within the medical and family planning communities to encourage women to use and to keep using IUDs. First, they were encouraged to view pain and bleeding as normal with IUD use. Women who were educated about this method knew that—according to medical professionals—endurance of "three or four months of pain" would eventually result in their having a "fine method of contraception and no more trouble." Furthermore, the experts believed that the less educated a woman was, the less pain she would endure. Education was said to be the key to "successful" IUD use. A woman's willingness to endure pain was thus an indication of her status and her success.[38]

For women injured by IUDs, the view that endurance of pain was a mark of education and social status posed a significant threat. When their endurance delayed their seeking treatment, their health and their lives could be threatened. There is some evidence that this threat was more intense for women of social privilege. One study showed that the wives of obstetrician-gynecologists had a higher rate of IUD use than the general population of contraceptors. Another study of women who used the Dalkon Shield showed that in the United States, the women who used the Dalkon Shield for the longest period of time after the dangers were known were the women with the highest levels of formal education.[39]

Among the women I interviewed there was one striking difference in the outcome of IUD injury. Women of privilege were able to purchase remedial care, including microsurgical procedures to repair damaged organs; in vitro fertilization to bypass the permanent damage to oviducts; and the services of world-renowned specialists for emergency medical intervention with problem pregnancies. The poorest women had the most extensive radical surgical procedures, including those known as total pelvic evacuations. All the women, however, regardless of social circumstances, were left with bodily damage that could cause them more difficulty in the future. For some women there was some surcease from pain and injury; for no injured woman was there a cure.

4 Gender and Sexuality

Most healthy women are capable of procreation for approximately forty years. An individual woman can experience approximately five hundred fertility cycles during those years. If a woman is exposed to the risk of pregnancy every time she is fertile, she could—if her body could withstand the strain—experience as many as fifty complete pregnancies. Procreative control is, therefore, an important issue for most women who are exposed to intercourse during extended periods of time during the forty or more years they are fertile. None of the women interviewed said that she would welcome unlimited pregnancies, but no one indicated that permanent sterility was an acceptable side effect of contraceptive use. The contradiction between the desire to control one's own procreative power and, at the same time, to protect it was a central issue raised by the women in this study.

Many of the women spoke of the importance of their ability to bear children. Heather had four children and a tubal ligation before she was 25 years old. She was not reconciled to the idea that she would never again bear a child. She said that her physician assured her that in all the years that he had been performing tubal ligations, no woman had ever subsequently become pregnant. Heather said the physician added, however, that "nothing's one hundred percent." It was hysterectomy that Heather feared would make her infertility "definite." She said:

> Part of me feels—that one of our greatest gifts is to have children—something that we have that—men don't have. I don't mean to say that women are just put on earth only to have offspring—but a man performs in his way and a woman performs in hers. If that part were taken away from me, I'd just feel that I wouldn't be as whole. I'd feel—that what I was put here partially for—as a woman—was taken away, and that I'd be less of a person—that it was so *definite* and I'd feel so *empty*.

Anna expressed similar feelings in speaking of her infertility: "To be able to give life—with someone you love deeply—is so much at the center of what I—as a woman—am equipped to do—and if I cannot do that I am *dry* and *barren* and *empty* in there—and I just don't want to live."

Nina was a mother of six who said that her children *were* her life. To Nina, the termination of fertility seemed like a kind of death. She said that she had once gone to a hospital to have a tubal ligation. She was on a stretcher, ready to be taken to the operating room, when her tears convinced her physician that she did not want the operation. Asked in the interview what her tears had been about, Nina replied, "It's like your life—your reproductive life—is over." Nina never had the tubal ligation.

The similarities between the sentiments expressed by Heather, Anna, and Nina indicate that gender to some extent transcends the boundaries of social class. Heather and Nina were both socially disadvantaged. Heather had left high school to have her first child, and never earned a diploma; Nina had taken some college courses, but was a single mother supporting six small children on a social welfare budget. Both Heather and Nina frequently referred in their interviews to economic hardships. Anna was the most socially privileged woman interviewed. She made it clear that financial concerns had been of little consequence in her life, even in her transatlantic quest for a means to overcome her infertility. Anna held a Ph.D. and had taught at an elite university during the time that her infertility caused her to think of suicide as a rational response to her pain. Despite the dramatic differences in their social circumstances, there was no difference in the passion with which each of these women expressed the linkage, for them, between life and reproductive capacity.

Anna expressed the contradiction that her need to control her procreative power had generated in her own life. As a young single woman attending college, she thought of her procreative power solely as something she had to curb. Anna stated with candor that she had been the "perfect dupe" when she purchased her Dalkon Shield. She said, "We fit together—women like me and the Robins company—we fit together perfectly. I was not even conscious that I was fertile—it was just not an issue for me. But the whole thing could have happened anyway, because people need birth control, even if they're fertility-conscious."

The women I interviewed often expressed their need for birth control with a sense of desperation. Ursula had two children when she was interviewed. She said that she had grown to love her children after they were born, but there had been a time in her life when she did not like children, and she had dreaded the idea that she might ever have to be a mother. Effectiveness had been her first concern when choosing a contraceptive method. She said, "I liked anything that would allow me not to get pregnant at the time." Safety was secondary in Ursula's assessment of contraceptives. Discussing her motivation for choosing an IUD, Ursula said, "At that point I wasn't really looking for, for *lots* of information on IUDs or birth control, all I knew was that I wanted a—a something that was reasonably safe and reasonably effective—and I thought—at the time that IUDs would do that—and they did, I mean they were real effective for me, *I didn't get pregnant.*"

The words *safe* and *effective* were often paired in women's discussion of birth control methods. At times the words were used interchangeably to refer to a method's ability to prevent pregnancy. Donna said that she decided to use the pill when she was eighteen because she believed it was the safest way to guard against pregnancy. Acknowledging that side effects were not being discussed at that time, Donna implied that by "safest" she meant that the pill was most effective in preventing pregnancy.

Theresa expressed the same concern. She said, "I had [my second child] and decided that two kids was great and that was *probably* all that I wanted to have. But I had been taking the pill before the birth of my *first* child, *nothing* between the first and *second,* and I realized that this nursing was not going to keep me safe *forever* as I had not been safe after the birth of my first, so—I—asked them—well, I think I did not *ask,* it was a matter of—them providing the information, but I would have asked at some point." Theresa said that if she had a daughter, she would tell her "not to expect—that—you're going to be *safe,* because that's *stupidity.*" Asked in what sense she meant safe, she replied, "Not becoming pregnant."

Melissa also used the word *safe* in reference to method effectiveness. She said, "I was told—I—I'm pretty sure I was told that, that the diaphragm, you know, there was—holes? Or that, you know, I'd heard stories of women forgetting to use it or, this or that and—it just seemed to me like from everything I heard I felt like this [using an IUD] is a safe way to do it and this is, and you won't get any problems with it and it would be easy—and I mean this was the part that was emphasized to me that this was an easy way to *do* it."

Women who had used IUDs referred to both safety in preventing pregnancy and safety as freedom from bodily harm when they explained their choice of method. Thirteen women had used oral contraceptives before they used an intrauterine device. Many of these women switched because of side effects from the pill. Mary had a series of ministrokes; Gretchen said she had unpleasant effects reminiscent of early pregnancy, including nausea; Nina became pregnant while using oral contraceptives, although she was certain that she never failed to take a pill. Olivia stopped taking birth control pills in order to get pregnant, and she did get pregnant "within days" after stopping the pills. She decided not to resume her use of the pill after her child was born because, she said, "I knew that I could get pregnant very easily if I missed a pill, so I decided to take the IUD, because I'm a very forgetful person and I'm always in a rush."

Valerie recalled an episode of sudden visual disturbances while taking oral contraceptives.

> I was shopping. I was talking to a friend, and I was looking at her—all of a sudden I could not see her, and just like a circle, like they used to have on—not the "Twilight Zone," but one of the others—where they block the middle of the TV, and then you can just see the outside, that's all I could see—and—I just kept blinking, and I kept thinking, "How am I going to get home?" It may have lasted about two minutes, but it seemed like a long time. And when it went away I said, "Forget it, I'm not taking the pill any more," and I just stopped.

Valerie rejected traditional methods of birth control, a decision based on her mother's experience. Valerie recalled, "My mother said with us— each one of us—there was something. I think [with] one of us there was the rhythm method, and she got pregnant; one was—the rubber—and she got pregnant; and one was—the diaphragm." Valerie wanted an effective method. She said that at the time that she chose the Dalkon Shield, an unplanned pregnancy would have meant disaster. She explained,

"My son wasn't planned either. It would have brought a lot of feelings; I might even have had an abortion. I feel bad for my son sometimes, because I really didn't—enjoy him—like I should have. I got married three days after graduation from high school. And then in November, I had my son. That's a really bad way to start a marriage, there's no doubt about it."

In response to the question, "Did you use anything [for birth control] before you got married?" Valerie said, "No. No. No, as a matter of fact, I didn't. I guess I was lucky for a little while, anyway." Asked, "Do you have any idea why you didn't?" she answered, "Um—just too lazy, I guess. First of all—it would have been more readily available for him, versus me. Um—and I just—I don't know. I guess being a kid you're in the heat of passion, why bother, you know, you're not going to get pregnant, and then before you know it—you are, and then you gotta deal with it." In response to the question, "Why would it have been more readily available to him?" Valerie responded, "Because—he could go to the drugstore and get rubbers. As opposed to me—I'd have—then I think you had to get permission from your parents to get an examination, as well as any kind of birth control—O.K.—I don't think it was as—confidential as it is today."

Francine was another woman who stressed that an early unplanned pregnancy had powerfully influenced her choices of contraceptive methods for the rest of her life. Francine learned that she was pregnant in 1955. She had successfully used the rhythm method for a year before it failed. When it did fail:

> It was devastating. It was probably the most difficult thing I've ever gone through in my life. I was a senior in high school. I would have been valedictorian of my class. I dropped out—of school—at my mother's request—three months before graduation. I was sixteen. It was devastating because I had already been accepted at two colleges. I had scholarships all lined up. Everybody was devastated; teachers were devastated, my friends, and my family. It was just a very difficult, difficult thing.

Francine was so determined to avoid another unplanned pregnancy that she and her husband often "doubled up" on methods. Even when she

used an IUD, Francine said that they also used a diaphragm with spermicide or a condom with spermicide at midcycle, to be "doubly sure that
there would be no more mistakes."

Francine discussed the options that she remembered having as a teenager in the 1950s:

> When I was in high school, methods that would have been available to a high
> school girl—um—there would have been none. Condoms were available to
> men. It's—I doubt that I would have been able, even if I had gone to a doctor, I
> doubt if a doctor would have prescribed—a diaphragm—although I didn't
> even know what a diaphragm was, I didn't even know they existed. I didn't
> know what they were. That was probably the most common method *women*
> were using then. Condoms for men. Rhythm was about the only method
> available—calendar rhythm. There were no devices and things that I knew of,
> except the diaphragm, and I didn't even know of the diaphragm until—after I
> was married my mother finally told me about—the diaphragm that she had
> been using for *years*. But I never knew what it was. Because no one had ever
> discussed those things with me. So I had no contraceptive education at *all*—
> when I was growing up.

Francine added, "What I mainly found out about sex I learned—by
having sex with my boyfriend, and that's how I learned."

Referring to her first pregnancy, Francine said that she "carried a lot
of guilt about that for a lot of years." Francine is now a health educator,
and she finds that some of the problems she experienced still apply to
young women today. She said, "I was ambivalent, because the social
messages are still the same: NICE GIRLS DON'T DO IT!"

Olivia also remembered knowing little about birth control when she
was young, but she thought that the situation for young women today
was much improved: "Back in the Dark Ages, I'll say—the time when I
was married—a lot of things were kept—from women as far as birth
control. As you can see by my age, I had my son when I was seventeen.
The pill wasn't available to single unmarried girls—in those days. Um—
and it's basically—like I'm so thrilled today that women have so many—
rights, which we always *had* but we just never voiced our opinion and
say, 'We want to know—what you're *doing* to us.' "

Asked what she might have told her daughter about birth control, Olivia said:

> We've talked a lot. My fear is that I remember how I was at fourteen, so I want to lock her in the closet. Even—well, I've had a lot of talks with my son, because he's seventeen and even though he's not dating and I'm a little less worried about him—the hard problem now is I'm born again, and—my beliefs and ideas have changed. And the belief is no sex before marriage. And it's a *little* hard to live up to, but I'm not dating and it's easy. My daughter, she feels the same way right now—that you shouldn't have sex before marriage—and you know, she's a real toughy and I'll say, "What would you do if a guy approached you?" and she says, "Well, I'd probably deck him," and I said, "Well, what if you really felt you were truly in love" because at sixteen I thought I *was.* I ended up luckily *marrying*—unluckily or luckily marrying the man who—I was engaged to and I got pregnant with, but, um, I talked to her a lot, and—well, *tonight*—I told her where I was going, and we were talking about IUDs and the pill, and she asked about the diaphragm, and—I told her as much as I know myself. And—I just said that—the *day* that she *decides*—um—that she wants to have sex, that [sigh] even though good girls aren't supposed to plan it and take protection—they both, um—I'm *positive* they both know that I got pregnant, and they saw what happened to my life so—I told her I'd take her to the doctor and discuss what's best. Because once you start you don't stop.

Olivia said she had also counseled her best friend's fifteen-year-old sister who was sexually active:

> She said she wasn't using any protection—yet the guy point-blank told her, "If you get pregnant, please don't let me know, I couldn't handle it!" And I said, "And you still want to *sleep* with this man?" And I—you know—and, you know—that's the type of thing that these girls go through—"Oh well, not me—I can't get pregnant." Well—yes you can! You know, so we had a really long talk. And I told her I'd even take her to Planned Parenthood, or something. Because I said I'm not going to tell you to stop because—it's too *late.* But I hope that when you *do* break off with this boy, that you go back to—*pretending* that you're a virgin again. And holding back.

Asked what method she might suggest a sexually active young girl use, Olivia said, "Right now I feel like I'd use the pill. Because I wouldn't trust—the male partner at all. They have all sorts of excuses about rubbers. And like, 'Well, if you don't climax you won't get pregnant.' Or, 'If you stand on your . . .' you know, they still *have* all these *stupid wives'* tales. And it gets me so angry. Well, I get very angry to see anybody *today* who gets pregnant by accident—*deserves* it. Because there are so many methods that's available."

The subject of men's responsibility for birth control was raised many times in the interviews. Several women said that they thought men should take more responsibility, and that more methods should be developed for men. Nina said, "Maybe they'll succeed in a program for men. I am not a feminist, but I think that it's about time that men had equal responsibility in things like this." Valerie said, "I'd personally like to see them do something for men. Let them take all this and that, you know— action. Let them be the ones, you know, that don't produce—fertile sperm—or whatever. It's kind of—unfair—that it's always up to the woman—to take precautions. I mean, it does take two—there are prophylactics—but, I mean—I think that women have enough to take care of. I'd like to see something done for the guys, personally."

Heather voiced the same concern: "It seems like women have to go through the pain, all the months of carrying the babies, all the changes in their systems—and if I chose that I wasn't ready to get pregnant again, then the least he could do was carry some of the responsibility—without—his is *external,* you know. And I thought, 'That's the least he could do' to—help carry the responsibility—or our *choice* in the responsibility of whether or not—our choice. He could do that much for me."

Heather's husband never shared her point of view about his responsibility to share in procreative control. Heather explained, "There was a lot of times when he intended on—him using condoms, and you get into the—situation—and you don't feel like stopping, or—suddenly you realize that you're out of them, you know, and—you just say, 'Forget it.'" For Heather, the material consequences of being out of condoms became life-threatening. Her third and fourth pregnancies were difficult. Her third child was born two months premature and had to have many weeks of intensive care. The child has learning disabilities related to oxygen deprivation after birth. Heather nearly lost her fourth child in the sixth month of pregnancy; she had a difficult delivery at term. The child sustained no apparent damage, but Heather was warned by her physician that any subsequent pregnancies would endanger her own life and would most likely result in miscarriage.

Heather discussed her struggle with her husband over which of them would undergo sterilization, once it was clear that she could safely sustain no more pregnancies:

> I felt that—if I didn't want any more kids, then he could get it done. It was cheaper. It was done in the office and he could go home. With me, it could set me back. After delivering a baby, I feel that's enough, do I have to go on? This argument went on for quite a while. You know, their manlihood steps in, and their pride, and they feel, I guess—I don't know how they look at it. They don't want anyone touching it—you know—that's *their* area. But every Tom, Dick, and Harry can look at us, you know. So, he kind of won—that it be me and not him. That was a relief to him. So, I was a little resentful about it.

Heather had a tubal ligation within days of delivering her fourth child. She said her heart stopped while she was under anesthesia, and the hospital staff had some difficulty reviving her. Within a year she had to return to the hospital for a second operation, after her physician discovered that she had developed a pelvic infection following the tubal ligation.

Heather told a story about deer hunting that illustrated the larger context of gender relations in her family informing the struggle over procreative control:

> Well, you want to hear something stupid, I can explain something recently, when we were tracking a deer my husband hit. It was a doe, O.K.? And they couldn't find the blood trail. I was standing on the last—blood—they had found. And I'm sitting there, and—I was originally—standing, which makes you taller than a deer, O.K.? So I squatted down. And I'm looking—the woods is a lot different when you see [it at] the eye level of a deer, you know. And I was thinking, "If I was a *female*—deer—and I was getting away from someone that—I was hurt—and my—I know I was being tracked, you know, someone was on my trail, where would I go?" And I was looking around and I seen— briars—you know, a thick patch, but it was open a little bit. And I thought, "I'd go right over there."
>
> Well, these guys couldn't find any blood, and I kept saying, "Look over there," and they weren't listening to me. I didn't want to move, 'cause I was

standing on the last spot of blood they had found. And I said, "Look over there." Finally, someone listened to me. And that's where it was. That happened three times while we were out there. It's just *instinct* to me."

Asked what it was about the deer following that particular path that she associated with the deer being female, Heather answered:

> Good question. Well, the deer, like the buck—always stays behind—he sends the female—and the babies—ahead of him. If they get hurt—he's safe, you know. I mean, there's male chauvinists in animals, too. And—to me, a female knows how to protect her young—quicker—than—whatever you be, human or animal or whatever mammal—than a man would. I—I don't know, I guess, men were tracking her, you know—and if I was a female deer—I—maybe I shouldn't say "female," maybe I should just say "deer," but it just seems like the buck makes a lot of mistakes—*without* the *help* of the *does*. You know, when they go out to feed in the open spots, they always send the female first. And it seems to me the female would use—use her head more, you know, and head in where *she* feels safest. And a buck without her would not know what to do. They'll—tend to go in circles. They lose their—bounds. And the females seem to get away better. So, I just feel that we're the same way, too.

Heather gave an example to illustrate the connection she was making between "female instincts" in deer and in humans. She said that her husband had an affair, and she turned to her father for advice. Her father blamed the affair on Heather and on the other woman, not on Heather's husband. He explained that men were not accountable for their actions, or reactions, when tempted by women. Heather, he claimed, needed to be a better wife so that maybe the next time a woman tempted her husband he would be able to resist. He said that men sometimes "get put in positions they can't get out of" because "that thing down there has no conscience."

Heather said:

> That's their excuse to me why men have affairs! If I was approached by a man, and I picked up—our *instincts* tell us they have feelings for us—I *certainly* know how to get out of it, and I wouldn't be falling into it, unless that's what I wanted, you know. That—stinks for an excuse! I was told a man can love his wife and still have an affair. Well—that's not what my morals are. That's not what I feel a *relationship*—should be. And if it was me, my *instincts* would tell me differently. I would *never* be put into that position. And it seems like, "Well, a

lot of men get put in positions they can't get out of." Well, why can't they? You know, why does a woman stop to think about *their* feelings, about their *husbands,* about their *children,* about their own true feelings before they *do?* *They* just *do* it, and then suffer for it later, you know. That stinks!

Pressed to clarify what she meant when she called what she was describing "instincts," Heather said

I don't know—do you feel that it's instincts? I don't know. Maybe it's part of my—*my* way of looking at life, at what it should be. I seem very old-fashioned. Today, in this world, it's easy come, easy go with marriages, relationships. What happened to the good old-fashioned way of when you say "I do" it's for truly it, you know. Not that affairs didn't happen in those days, but it seemed like—it was a lot less divorce—and violence—and more concrete—family. When you get down to family, that was it. And that's what I believe. But it don't seem like anybody else does around me. And I label that as—womanly instincts. I'm comfortable with family. I'm more comfortable with family than I would be alone, maybe even alone career-oriented. If all I had was a career, I don't think I'd be happy either. Just like now, all I have is my family, and I'm not happy either, you know. I want both. I want it all—and it's hard.

Like Heather, Gretchen felt that responsibility for birth control had fallen exclusively to her by her husband's default.

When I decided to have the Dalkon Shield put in I had just had my second baby, and it was at my six-week checkup. I was twenty-one and I had my second child. I knew I didn't want any more, and I had tried the birth control pill, in between my first and my second one. I felt really awful when I was on it—I felt just like I was pregnant, with morning sickness and everything else. So, I really just didn't—I thought that was the best thing to use at the time.

One of my sisters had had one put in, and it seemed to be O.K. for her. And so I just thought I would try the same thing. The other reason I didn't want to try the birth control pill was because a friend had—at that same time—a friend had had a stroke. She was on the pill, and she was younger than I was—she was 20—and she had a stroke from the pill. And I just thought between the way I felt when I was on it, and what was happening to her, I didn't want to do that again.

There was not a choice of different IUDs, that was just the one that the doctor was using. I had heard other people say at that time that they had a different kind, but it wasn't like, "Well, would you like this one, or would you like that one?" It was just like that was the IUD that this doctor was using. And—because I didn't want the pill—that was the only option. I just saw it as something I should try. I never knew that there could be dangers with it. And it just seemed like it was harmless. It really did.

The insertion process was *very, very* painful. And I remember it was terrible—he had a student and he was showing her how an IUD was put in. I wasn't crazy about having someone there observe the whole thing. But I remember how painful it was—it really was—it was painful. Whatever they used to measure the cervix or something like that, it was just really painful. And then when he inserted it something must have gotten torn, because he had to use something to make it stop bleeding. And then he said that I had to lay there for an extra amount of time before he would let me sit up. But I remember being—afraid—because I knew that whatever happened when he put it in wasn't normal. But he sent me home, and it was uncomfortable for a couple of days, and then it seemed to subside.

It seemed to work O.K. for me for at least two or three years. And then when I went for a regular checkup he just told me, "I'm going to take this out." I wasn't crazy about having it taken out because it wasn't giving me any trouble, and I knew I would have to figure out what I was going to do then. But he was just real insistent that it should be taken out. He recommended that we take that one out, wait a few months, and then put another kind in. It was after the publicity had hit the newspapers.

He wanted me to try a diaphragm, and I did try but I couldn't—it was a real humiliating exerience—because I couldn't get it in right. I was in his office and he said, "You're *not* going to leave here until that is in correctly!" But he would just leave his office and leave me in there, and I was in tears because I didn't know what I was doing wrong. He would come in and say, "It's not in right!" and then he would leave. I didn't know why I wasn't putting it in right. Finally—I think it was just out of pure coincidence—I did put it in right and he let me leave. But then when I went home I said, "How reliable is this? How am I going to know if it's in right or if it's not in right?" So I figured that it wasn't going to work, because I wasn't sure at *all* how to put it in right.

I really felt comfortable with an IUD, because I knew it would stay in until I did otherwise. My second IUD was the Cu-7. I knew what I was getting into when I had it put in. I wasn't looking forward to it at all. But it wasn't as bad as the first one being put in, and I didn't have any noticeable problems. Because it worked for me, I just thought it was O.K.—I wasn't having any trouble with it. I had it in for between three and four years. When I went in for a regular checkup to the doctor he said that he was going to take it out. It was the same as the other time, it wasn't like a decision that was made between the two of us, he just said, "I think that it would be best if I took it out." So, I think that through the years he probably realized how damaging they could be. But I was actually kind of angry, because it was like—"This is working O.K. for me, and now I don't have anything. Now I'm back to the same old thing. The same old

thing—what do you use?" And so we were back to using condoms. That went
on for maybe a year or so. And then after enough complaining from my
husband about using the condoms, I was calling different doctors to see which
doctor would put in an IUD. I did a lot of phoning, because there were really
very few doctors who were putting in IUDs in 1981.

But I finally found a doctor. I called and I said, "Does he still believe in
using IUDs?" and they said yes. So, I made an appointment with him. The first
thing he did was take me into his office and he went—at least for an hour—on
why I shouldn't have an IUD put in. His first thing—he was really pro-pill—
and he told me that if I used the pill, my facial hair would be much improved.
And I thought, "Why are you talking about my facial hair?" It was the last thing
that I—the last thing in the *world* . . . I mean you can deal with that with other
ways than using the birth control pill! To me it was just crazy.

But—his biggest objection to the IUD wasn't that it's dangerous—he went
on to a moral thing about, "Do you know what an IUD does, how it works?" I
said, "It makes it so that the egg can't implant itself." And he said, "It's not just
an *egg!* It's a *fertilized* egg!" And he went on this whole thing about how it was the
same as an abortion. And to me it was terrible, because it was like saying to you
that you've had an IUD in for all those years and you were committing
abortion after abortion after abortion. His whole argument was really moral.

Even though I was there to have an IUD put in, I was really apprehensive
about the whole thing because I didn't—I knew it could be very painful. So I
really had to talk myself into going. But it was just something that I said, "Well,
I've got to do this. We've got to do something else, I don't want to keep
listening to the whole thing about the condom." So—I finally said to the
doctor, "If I was going to have an IUD put in, I certainly wouldn't have you put
it in anyway!" Because he was just so—*mean* about the whole thing. Here I was,
I wasn't crazy about it anyway because I knew it was going to be painful, and I
didn't want this person who had just got through yelling at me for an hour
telling me I was morally wrong. . . . I mean, he finally said, "I'll put one in if
you want." But it was like, "Sure!" I mean, I didn't even feel comfortable
having the doctor even—examine me. But I did. I stayed.

I knew that the only thing I was going to leave with was the pill. And that was
it. I remember leaving, paying $120 or something. I was totally humiliated. I
ended up leaving with something I really didn't feel was good for me. I wasn't
crazy about taking it. I never really felt comfortable taking it. But I did take it
the whole time that the prescription was good for, but I said, "I'll be darned if
I'm going back to that doctor and paying him to—you know. I just didn't want
anything to do with him. Now I'm back to square one again, because I'm
without anything—with no doctor. So it just seems like a vicious circle.

Valerie, who had originally said that she wanted men to share responsibility for birth control, later qualified those initial remarks. She said that even if a contraceptive pill were developed for men,

> Women would still be afraid. Being—you know—being able to get pregnant, or the guy saying, "Yeah, I'm on the pill," and then not being on the pill. I mean, I think men are a little leery, but they're apt to believe a woman about being on the pill—or some kind of contraceptive. So they'll say, "O.K., it doesn't matter." But, I don't know, men are funny that way. They don't—it's O.K. for us to take the risks, but they don't want to. I think sometimes it's their macho ego. They feel it's going to be deflated by being—it's the same as having a vasectomy. There's a lot of men who refuse—it's gonna—*interfere* with their manlihood. They won't be able to perform.

Concern for the "macho egos" of men was reflected in the words of Dr. Robert Kistner in a 1969 article in the *Ladies' Home Journal*:

> It is generally accepted that the male is much more susceptible to psychological factors in his sexual activity than the female. His virility, sense of maleness, even his self-esteem are more closely allied to the sexual act than that of a woman. Impotence is far more debilitating psychologically to the male than frigidity is to the female. Although he usually plays the aggressor's role in sexual relations, he is extremely sensitive to even slight affronts to his masculinity. For all these reasons, it has been assumed that any method of contraception that diminished sperm count would create psychological problems for many men, leading to ego loss and impotence.[1]

Concern about alleged physical and psychological side effects of contraceptive products and procedures for men has delayed the marketing of several methods for many years. Gossypol, one such product, is a derivative of cottonseed oil. The substance was discovered in 1886, according to an article in *The Lancet,* but "no mention was made of its antifertility effect" until Chinese scientists made that claim in the 1950s. It was tested on 8,806 men in China beginning in 1972 and was found to be 99 percent effective. The substance caused a serious potassium deficiency in 0.75 percent of the men. It caused irreversible infertility in 10 to 20 percent. Because of these problems, the article predicted, Gossypol would not lead to the development of a widely marketed male contraceptive pill "in this century."[2]

In 1974 Dr. C. Alvin Paulsen was reported to have tested combinations of two synthetic hormones—one similar to progesterone and another similar to testosterone—on a group of a hundred men. A monthly injection was found to be highly effective, but return to fertility took several months after the medication was stopped.[3] The drug has never been marketed.

Several devices have been designed to block the vas deferens. Some resemble a plug made either of plastic or metal; others are thin wires of copper inserted into the vas. These devices are called IVDs or IVCDs (intravas devices, or intravas contraceptive devices). A "valve" that could be turned on and off was also tried.[4] These devices were designed in the hope of providing men with a form of contraception as effective as vasectomy, but reversible. None of these devices is commercially available at the time of this writing.

Francine said that her husband did cooperate in efforts to assure that no unplanned pregnancies occurred during their marriage. She said that he had been reluctant to buy condoms when they were teenagers, "not to use them, but to buy them." After the unplanned pregnancy and subsequent marriage, however, he shared the responsibility for birth control. Ultimately he had a vasectomy—when Francine was forty-one years old. Francine said:

> It was a burden I had always borne, ever since I was fifteen—every month was always, you know—wondering, will my period come, will it not; did the diaphragm slip this month or did it not; was the condom we used O.K. or wasn't it—or whatever. Just a constant worry, month after month, year after year after year. It built up to the point that he decided while I was away to have a vasectomy done, without consulting me. I was just overwhelmed with—with that, because it was such a wonderful gift he gave me. He gave me the gift of freedom, is what he did.

Francine had some ambivalent feelings about her husband's decision, however. She said, "I was thrilled in one way that he had taken the responsibility. But in another way—that still—left me—potentially able to get pregnant. If I had an affair—or if—he died—or we *divorced*, I would *still*, regardless of the circumstances—*I'm still vulnerable* to pregnancy and having to rely on *his* operation. That bothered me a great deal, because I've always taken great pride all my life in taking care of myself."

Ursula also had ambivalent feelings about birth control for men:

Basically, in my own situation, I have been almost 100 percent responsible for—birth control—in our family. I mean, it's either been me on the pill, or having an IUD. So, I think that sort of share-and-share alike might come in somewhere along the road for—for male birth control. It's sort of like doing housework. I don't like doing housework *either,* but it's nice to *share* it. So, when the responsibilities for birth control lie primarily with the woman, I think it would be nice to think that you could share it.

Ursula thought, however, that it would be difficult to develop a birth control product for men. She said, "It seems to me that, logically, it's much easier to prevent *one egg* from ovulating every month, than, you know, THOUSANDS AND MILLIONS OF SPERM, um, from being produced *every other day.* That might really be a silly prejudice on my part, and if I knew more—physiology and biology I might say that—it wouldn't be so difficult to do it—if someone really wanted to try—but it just seems to me that—they're a long way from doing anything, right now."

Before turning to Ursula's comments about vasectomy, let us consider her attitude about the risks associated with the methods she used. Ursula's family had a history of breast cancer, a fact that influenced her to switch from oral contraceptives to IUDs:

Basically I was happy with an IUD. I mean, *I* found them a lot better than taking birth control pills. I think if it hadn't been for the fact that I used them so long that I was getting a continual inflammation in my uterus which was— causing me to have my periods so *often*—I mean, twenty-one days is not—I mean, when you think that your period starts at day *one,* is going to last until day *nine* and then at day twenty-*two* you're going to have another period again—that's a pain in the neck. And that's what was happening."

Despite these problems, Ursula said, "You know, I was a pretty satisfied user of an IUD, without knowing what the risks were and yet not being affected by them at all. But, you know, I knew the risks were there, but I was willing to take them, for the convenience of the method." Pressed to explain what she believed the risks were that she had taken when she made the choice to use an IUD, she explained,

Well, I knew the chance of pelvic inflammatory disease was there. I felt like I was really not terribly at risk for that, because I had one—sexual partner. I knew there was a slight possibility that I would get pregnant—and I think that's *always* a problem with IUDs, 'cause then you have to—to worry about it being ectopic—an ectopic pregnancy. I knew there was some risk of, um—scarring—um, inflammation which would—might—increase the chances of being infertile. I can't remember anything else. I really wasn't worried about PID. I think at the time, I really wasn't worried about whether I would get pregnant or not, because it seemed like something I didn't want to have happen at the time, anyway. I didn't worry very much about becoming pregnant, I just figured I wouldn't be one of the, one in a hundred, or two in a hundred that it happened to. Again, I think I was willing to take an informed risk of doing that. I knew that there were problems all along with IUDs in terms of—pelvic inflammatory disease—again, you know, it always seemed to be limited with women who had multiple sexual partners, and that, again, was not—where I was coming from—so I wasn't worried about that.

I know a friend of mine which got pregnant with an IUD. I *knew* that happened. Again—you know—it probably happens to what? One out of a hundred women? Or something like that? You hope it's not you, and you hope it's not one of your friends—essentially—and, I think, that's all you can ask—is to ask—you know, is to make an informed decision. I mean, you know, there's so many things that can go wrong with so many drugs . . .

Ursula's assessment of the potential risks of vasectomy was inconsistent with her assessment of the risks in her own use of IUDs. However, her feelings about vasectomy risks were backed by reports in the medical literature, which linked the method with atherosclerosis and possible immunosuppression. She said, "I think my husband would be willing to have a vasectomy, but *I'm* not convinced that that's the safest way to go—ultimately. One—guy—did—a study on—vasectomies in rabbits, and they—definitely found autoimmune antibodies in the kidneys of rabbits who had been vasectomized. I'm not convinced that enough research has accumulated on vasectomies, to say that they're not going to be—that they're completely safe." Ursula added, "And except for the initial surgery and the risks that go with that, I—I think that tubal ligation *can* be fairly harmless. I mean, most of the people I know that have had it that truly *wanted* it—have not had *problems*."

Mary expressed no ambivalent feelings about turning over the responsibility for birth control to men. She very definitely wanted to maintain control over her own procreative power. For Mary, who had had open-heart surgery, a pregnancy could have fatal complications. She said, "I don't think we should rely on male birth control. It's my body. I will protect it. It's my body and if I don't want to have children, and I want to have sex, I will therefore do what is necessary. Not only that, but I can trust *myself.* You know—I don't want to put that responsibility in someone else's hands." Another consideration influenced Mary's attitude. She said, "In my—generation—if you got pregnant it was your fault. It was not his."

Many of the women interviewed equated the use of birth control with personal liberation. The pill was often cited as a revolutionary promise of almost 100 percent freedom from compulsory motherhood. Ursula said:

> I think birth control is a real *problem.* You know, it's just that in the *sixties* it seemed like the problem was going to be solved. And it's not. In fact, you're probably *worse*—well, you're not worse off, you're better off now, because— various birth control methods have been tested and we can make informed decisions. But, I think, you know, and the dosages of estrogen were too high and all that stuff—it's real hard. But I think it's a far more complicated—what do I want to say?—it's a lot more complicated to regulate the human *body*— even in that one system—than anyone anticipated it would be.

One of the effects of the advent of oral contraceptives had been the promise of increased efficacy. Another had been the promise of sexual spontaneity—the mechanics of birth control could be separated from the time and place of intercourse. By the time the Dalkon Shield became available, barrier methods had become unpopular. Several women voiced objections they had had to barrier methods when they chose an IUD. Megan recalled that condoms were, at that time, "a joke." Olivia said the diaphragm "bothered" her because it was "unromantic." Mary didn't like the use of the diaphragm because, she said, "That to me isn't freedom, it's another type of chain." Donna was more concerned that the diaphragm wasn't safe enough. By *safe,* she explained that she meant effective in preventing pregnancy.

Many physicians and scholars welcomed birth control methods that promised separation of sexual expression from the demands of contraceptive use. Dr. Alan Guttmacher described his idea of an ideal contraceptive:

> An ideal contraceptive method would have many requirements. It should be harmless, reliable, free of objectionable side reactions, inexpensive, readily

reversible, simple to use, and unlikely to impair full sexual satisfaction for either partner. A "coitally independent" contraceptive—a method applied at a time wholly dissociated from the sexual act so that a couple need not anticipate intercourse nor interrupt the process to achieve protection against impregnation—is more likely to allow full spontaneity and to permit full sexual satisfaction.[5]

Garrett Hardin voiced similar preferences:

The time of pill-taking is completely divorced from the time of love-making. There is no psychological interference here. There is no prevention of total mutual abandon. The necessary cautious forethought and the desirable gay abandon can coexist in the same person, because separated in time. This was the possibility created by the pill. It was this possibility that made both the rhythm method and the traditional contraceptive devices seem, by comparison, undesirable.[6]

Dr. Hugh J. Davis used this argument to promote IUDs in general and his Dalkon Shield in particular. He wrote, "Because of its many unique advantages, intrauterine contraception is proving to be an ideal method for an increasing number of women, providing a practical means of fulfilling man's ancient dream of separating sexual expression from involuntary reproduction."[7]

Apparently the availability of effective contraceptive methods caused other psychological problems for some men. In an article entitled "Tell Me Doctor: 'Why Did Birth Control Fail Me?'" Barbara Seaman disclosed the following: "Bernard Frankel, a Long Island clinical psychologist, says that a surprising number of men seem to fear that their wives would 'run around with other men' if they were not afraid of having a baby that might be hard to explain. He tells of one husband who went so far as to substitute aspirin for his wife's birth-control pills, because he suspected her of having a love affair with the man next door."[8] One of the "benefits" of IUD use was that it did not leave women vulnerable to this kind of subterfuge—a device worn internally could not be altered or easily removed without the woman's knowledge.

The high rate of effectiveness associated with oral contraceptives posed a problem for women who became pregnant while using that method. Oral contraceptive failure is typically thought to occur because a woman willfully or accidentally neglects to take the pill daily. But researchers are aware that antibiotic therapy or gastrointestinal illness can interfere with the contraceptive effect of the pill, causing unintended pregnancy in women who take the pills faithfully.[9] The myth persists, however, that pill failure is user failure, a factor that may influence some women to use other methods, like IUDs or injectable or implantable contraceptives, over which they have little control. Having relinquished control, they cannot be blamed for failure.

An IUD seemed like an ideal method of contraception to many women who were seeking an alternative to oral contraceptives and who didn't want to sacrifice the effectiveness or the freedom that the pill had promised. Several women said they liked using an IUD because they didn't have to "think about" or "worry about" it. Gretchen said, "It was convenient. Something I didn't have to think about."

Valerie explained that she had liked using the Dalkon Shield. She said, "I myself think the IUD is the laziest way. It's the easiest way as long as you don't have pain. It's easy, per se, I mean it's there, you don't have to worry about, 'Oh, I forgot to take the pill,' or you don't have to say, 'Stop, I have to put the lotion on my diaphragm, or the contraceptive gel, or the prophylactics.' It's there, you don't have to worry about it, you can go about your business."

Valerie mentioned the importance of the "sexual revolution":

The thing is I think nowadays, not so much this generation, but was it what?—in the early seventies?—midseventies?—it was that sexual revolution, you had to see how many people you could—sleep with in your lifetime, where it was really *bad,* and there was no reason for unwanted pregnancies, all right? Today—um—I think they're thinking a little more, "Well geez, should I really do it?" Um—I do think there's a little more options, but it still comes back to the same old thing—you know—in the back of your mind there's the first thing is you don't do it, then you don't have to *worry* about it.

Melissa had never used a method of contraception before she purchased her Dalkon Shield, as she had never been sexually active. Melissa's explanation of why she preferred an intrauterine device illustrated the tension between the ideology of sexual liberation and the more traditional mores that proscribed sexual activity for young single women.

Melissa said, "I was very relieved to have it and I felt a sense of freedom, and I thought, 'Oh, I don't have to worry about this thing.'" Asked what alternatives had been offered at the clinic where she purchased the Dalkon Shield, Melissa said, "I think I was pretty clear before—I think I had read enough beforehand on my own (I don't know where I got the literature). The whole thing in my memory—it was so long ago it's hard to remember—*but*—it just feels like, um, I must have known, because I was very clear that I wanted an IUD. I definitely didn't want the pill and I didn't want a diaphragm, so it was definitely my choice, when I walked in this is what I wanted." In response to the question, "Why didn't you want the pill?" Melissa answered, "I think I didn't want any telltale signs around that I was using birth control. So I think it was like embarrassment about—about being a sexual person. . . . I guess I was probably—it just *felt easier* to me to just deal with it. It was something you had just put in once and you don't have to worry about it again—so I *thought!*"

Nina chose an IUD for similar reasons. She said, "I thought that it was convenient, something I didn't have to think about." She had used the diaphragm before she decided to get the Dalkon Shield. In response to the question, "Did you like the diaphragm?" Nina answered, "No. It's inconvenient." She explained, "To have to plan ahead and to think about when you're going to have sex, and to, um, you know—I like the spontaneity."

Later in Nina's interview we discussed the subject of the diaphragm again. Nina's comments brought up the issue of women's sexual roles in relationship to the method of contraception chosen. Asked, "When you use birth control, what's the first thing that comes to mind when you're thinking about a method?" Nina answered:

> I guess effectiveness—and then I guess convenience. You know, the ease of using it. My brother and his wife have used spermicidal foam for years, and she hasn't had an unwanted pregnancy in that time, but I think it's inconvenient. My sister used that too for a long time and it worked out fine for her. . . . It's the planning on it, ahead of time. I'm not an organized person, and it was inconvenient for me to have to think, "Well, are we or aren't we?" And if we didn't then I would feel frustrated by having used it. I don't know.

With an IUD, then, Nina would always be prepared when her husband chose to have sex; and she would not be reminded that she had been prepared if he did not choose to have sex. Either way, with an IUD Nina "didn't have to think about" her sexuality.

IUDs allow sex without forethought and forethought without sex—a resolution to the conflict between liberation and traditional ideologies. That resolution had tragically ironic consequences for some women. Melissa, who remained involuntarily childless fifteen years after having the Dalkon Shield removed, did not know whether she would ever be able to bear a child. She knew that the acute pelvic inflammatory disease she suffered left her oviducts scarred to the extent that physicians warned her that she was susceptible to ectopic pregnancies, if she could become pregnant at all. Ironically, Melissa's Dalkon Shield served no practical purpose for much of the time that she had it. Melissa said, "Pretty soon after I got the Dalkon Shield I stopped being involved with the person I was involved with, so I was not being sexually active for most of the time that I had the Dalkon Shield."

Competing ideologies had another consequence for Anna. Anna said that when she learned that her use of the Dalkon Shield had left her infertile, "It felt at first like I was going to be punished for past sexuality." Anna had been tortured by thoughts that, had she not been such a rebel, her mother might have helped her by taking her to a better doctor. It was clear that for Anna, sexual activity at the time that she had the Dalkon Shield was itself a major part of the rebellion that left her estranged from her mother and feeling guilty for her own injuries and pain.

Mary made a comment that juxtaposed the choice of contraceptive method with another choice: the choice to engage in a mode of sexual expression with its own inherent risks. I interviewed Mary after I had taught a course in women's health and sexuality. I had overheard a conversation between two young women who were leaving the lecture hall after I spoke about the Dalkon Shield. One of the young women said to the other, "I never would have put one of those things into *my* body." I asked Mary how she would respond to that comment, and she quickly answered, "I would ask them what they *would* put in their bodies. I mean, you're talking about sexually—you're putting a *man* inside your body, plus his sperm. I mean, you're putting a strange piece of someone else's body in yours. So, you're saying that you couldn't put a Dalkon Shield in your body? Come on! Are your ears pierced?"

Mary was the only person interviewed who raised the point that heterosexual intercourse itself is of questionable safety for women. That fact is always implicit in the necessity to use contraception. Contraceptive use does not simply imply that sexual expression is anticipated—it implies that a particular form of sexual expression is anticipated. Vaginal-penile intercourse is the only form of sexual expression that requires contraception. If we accept the evidence available to us in the popular culture and in the work of professional sex researchers, it is clear that many persons engage in a variety of other forms of sexual expression.[10] Yet the ideology prevails that vaginal-penile intercourse is sex, and that abstinence from it—regardless of other forms of sexual expression that might be preferred—is abstinence from sex.

This ideology is so deeply entrenched that it is implicit even in the latest edition of the Boston Women's Health Collective's *The New Our Bodies, Ourselves,* which is a self-consciously antisexist women's health book. While abstinence is recognized in that book as a valid form of birth control, the word carries unfortunate implications.[11] Many people interpret the word *abstinence* as meaning affection without intercourse *and* without orgasm rather than as sex, including orgasm, without vaginal-penile contact. The implication that not to engage in one form of sexual expression is to abstain from sex altogether centralizes that one form of sexual expression as the norm against which all other forms are measured and found wanting.

Theresa made a comment about condoms that hinted at the danger inherent in vaginal penetration by a penis. To the question, "Did you ever consider using condoms?" she answered, "I think we tried that once, you know, I was nervous about it—it was a foreign body. I don't think that I felt comfortable about it." In response to the question, "Did you feel that it was not a reliable method of birth control, or was it the condom itself that bothered you?" she said, "I don't think I wanted anything artificial there—now that's interesting because the IUD certainly is [pause], but the IUD once inserted was *there* and somewhat stable I guess. [Pause.] I did not feel comfortable—with a condom." Theresa's recognition of the condom as "a foreign body" was perhaps one step away from recognition of the penis as a foreign body.

Heather raised an issue that made it clear that for her, sexual intercourse was not always a matter of choice. Heather rejected the pill and the IUD because her mother had suffered uterine cancer and her sister had been injured by the Dalkon Shield. She did not want to risk injury from those methods. Barrier methods also frightened her, so she had used only calendar rhythm, and that without success. She explained, "It was hard for me to pinpoint the bad times because I was never regulated. But—I used my better judgment at times, and, you know, it pretty much worked better than—the other. It was too easy to say don't worry about condoms, you know, 'Forget it.' " Rhythm was a problem sometimes, she said, because, "You know—if he wasn't—men are men, when they want it, they want it, you know. And he didn't always—ask."

Her physician was not pleased with Heather's decision not to use the pill. Heather's explanation of her physician's attitude betrayed her own feelings about sexuality. Heather said, "She felt that was more ignorance to—to sex, and the, you know—the whole ordeal—than it was making a logical or sensible decision."

For Valerie, fear of pregnancy and her inability to use the pill or IUD made sexual intercourse less than satisfying. In response to the question, "What are you using now for birth control?" Valerie said, "As my girlfriend's mother used to say, her husband's a good conductor—'he pulls out on time.' Which is—which he does—and I don't really think it's a good method of birth control. For many reasons—one, I mean, there is a chance that I could get pregnant, but we've been married for like—almost eight years, and that hasn't happened. But it can be frustrating for me. I don't really—appreciate—not that it's—I don't know how to explain. I just—feeling that there's—something missing."

Asked why they had not used condoms, Valerie said, "We've tried it and we weren't too keen on the rubbers. I didn't like them—I mean I—I myself thought they were kind of painful. I don't know whether I wasn't—

lubricated enough—during, you know, the course of relations. I—I just didn't like them. I thought they were uncomfortable. Almost like they dragged." Valerie had also rejected the diaphragm. She said, "I've used the diaphragm and—I had no problem with it, O.K. The only thing is that—my husband said that he *could* feel it a little, but which wasn't dis-com . . . discomfort to him—however—there was a time when I thought I got pregnant. And ever since then even when I have the diaphragm in he'll still pull out. So I just don't bother any more, I figure why should I?"

There were ironic consequences to using IUDs to make intercourse possible and "safe." For at least two of the women interviewed, IUD injuries ultimately made intercourse painfully difficult. Natalie said, "One night after having intercourse, like five minutes later, I got this really, really bad pain. And I started to cry—that's how bad it got. I didn't know what to do. I couldn't take the pain. I was grabbing my lower abdomen and crying, lying on the floor." After that, Natalie said, "I was afraid to have sex. I worried when I did, and I was careful, I was paranoid that any move on his part would make me hurt." The effect of Natalie's injuries went beyond the pain during intercourse. Orgasm became impossible. Natalie said, "You know how sometimes you have intercourse that you burn a lot of calories? I don't, and I say, 'Don't even try it, please. Not with me.' And it has to be very gentle. I can't have—orgasms—and I think it's because of that—because I'm afraid to—I'm so scared I start to hurt. And I never had that before the IUD, and it's something that has got progressively worse. I really feel like all my insides are rotting. That's what I've felt—like all my insides are rotting . . ."

Olivia said her marriage broke up at about the same time she had her Dalkon Shield removed. During the last year of her marriage intercourse had become painful for her. She said, "I—was having a lot of pain while I was having sex with my husband. . . . And, it got to this point where—my husband couldn't enter me, without me screaming—and pulling away."

It was clear from the interviews that stoicism was considered to be a desirable response to pain and suffering for women. The women who had experienced childbirth no doubt had that ideology reinforced for them during that experience. Women are expected to endure childbirth "without pain" or, at the very least, without complaint. The language of modern childbirth instruction is a language of social control—women are expected to exercise self-control of a caliber sufficient to overcome or to conceal the physical discomfort—the pain—involved in birthing a baby.[12] For many women who have gone into the delivery room determined to act "correctly" and thus to earn the respect and admiration of the presiding authorities, this ideology has turned out to be a myth and a cruel hoax.

The women interviewed were willing to endure what they often described as an "excruciating" degree of pain in order to control their procreative power effectively and still engage in sexual intercourse. All of the women interviewed who used IUDs were asked what it was like for them to use that method. Most described IUD insertion as painful. Nancy said that the pain was so bad that she "almost went off the table at the other end, it was excruciating." Nancy's motivation to use a method that would assure maximum protection against pregnancy was proved by her return for a second insertion attempt after the first painful attempt proved impossible.

Olivia described her experience with having the Dalkon Shield put into her uterus: "It was painful. And I remember—I'm brave. I don't yell at pain or anything. But I told him I'd like to see *him* get on the table and let me do something like that to *him*. I've been through—an operation and having two kids, but it definitely was uncomfortable. I mean, I didn't scream and kick and they didn't have to tie me down like I hear some girls are—overly—dramatic. But it wasn't any picnic."

Valerie's comments epitomized the response of women to the pain of IUD use: "It was painful, but—tolerable—let's put it that way. I felt the pain was worth it—the, um, you know—not getting pregnant." Anna echoed those sentiments, saying that she "paid her dues to the thing" by enduring the pain, and she wanted to "reap the benefits."

Nine of the women interviewed suffered severe illnesses presaged by pain that the women tried to tolerate. Donna said that despite the fact that she would have "awful pain and cramps" and that "two weeks of every month were taken up" with her menstrual period, she "stuck with" the Dalkon Shield for two years before deciding that "it wasn't worth it, any more." She said: "[I] was determined that, you know—I mean, this is what I needed to do, and I was going to suffer through the pain and it would be *over,* and I would be O.K." Donna's pain was not over even after her Dalkon Shield was finally removed. She had an ectopic pregnancy that ruptured twice, seriously threatening her life, requiring extensive surgery, and ending a planned and much desired pregnancy. Donna's fertility was restored after expensive and painful reconstructive surgery to repair her oviducts. At the time of the interview, more than ten years after removal of the Dalkon Shield, Donna still suffered pain from pelvic adhesions.

Melissa said that she tried to be "stoical" about her pain because she was "depending on [the Dalkon Shield] for birth control." She described her illness:

> It was sort of like this thing that came on very gradually, where I—I was just exhausted, and my legs—would ache—I would like, walk upstairs, and the *bones* would ache. It was—it was really a horrible—experience. Then it was bizarre—it was a bizarre illness. Then I started *bleeding* and I was bleeding for—what I thought was my period—and it never stopped. And I was bleeding for—several weeks—and—at the time I was, I guess I was just being stoical and—felt like—"Oh, a woman shouldn't complain about their bodies, and this is just—I've been told that sometimes women have irregular periods, and, if you bleed a little extra, that wouldn't—don't worry about it." So, I thought that it was one of those quirky things, and sooner or later it would be fine. And then I finally decided, "Well, this has really been going on too long, and I should go to the doctor next week and make an appointment." And then, I think it was Sunday, I was just going about my business, and doing housework or something, and I was all of a sudden just doubled over with pain—and it was excruciating *abdominal* pain that I was just all of a sudden on the *floor,* and I think I *crawled* into—I was living in a house where several other people were— and I just asked for—another woman was there—and I asked for some help, and she called the emergency room. So, some friends took me to the hospital. I had to wait a long time of course. Meanwhile, I was in excruciating pain, and the doctor said, "Well, we think you have—an ectopic pregnancy, a tubal pregnancy," and he said, "It *may* be because of the IUD, and *maybe* we should take it out." But he said, "Do you want it out?" And I said, "Well, I don't want it out if I don't have to, if that's not the *problem* I don't want it out." Because I had been *depending* on it for birth control. So I said, "O.K., we'll leave it in then."

Two weeks later the physicians removed Melissa's Dalkon Shield, after concluding that she had a pelvic infection caused by the device.

Theresa also became severely ill while using the Dalkon Shield. Her husband doubted the authenticity of her illness:

> I remember going to a bicentennial celebration . . . and feeling *very, very* ill, as if I were going to pass out, and feeling feverish and going home and pro-ceed[ing] to feel sicker and sicker, and I had company—my in-laws were there—and it was very uncomfortable, not being able to take care of them and so forth, and trying to *fake* feeling O.K. . . . I just got worse the next day and the fever was *so* bad I *did* call the doctor. I went *in* and he removed the shield. I think he knew, immediately, that it was causing the problem, because I had severe cramping and I was not susceptible to cramping when I had my period. So he removed it and sent me home and gave me some antibiotics and said if I didn't feel better to call him; and a day or two later I woke up and I could not—remain still, I was shaking so badly. My husband had a board meeting that morning. He was convinced that I was not that sick. I told him I was, and board meeting or no board meeting he was going to take me to the emergency room, which the doctor said I should do if I felt worse, and he did, immediately, and I was there for—eight days.

Theresa said her husband told her, "You would pick the day I had a board meeting."

Melissa related the story of a woman she had met whose situation illustrated the linkages between personal relationships, contraceptive use, the isolation of women in cases of contraceptive injury, and the role of physicians in perpetuating gender roles that put women with IUDs at particular risk:

> Just last weekend I met a woman who had—the Dalkon Shield—probably ten years ago, also. She was telling her story, of what happened to *her*. She had the Dalkon Shield for two years, and had incredible profuse bleeding. She was very concerned about it—she said her first period after she got the Dalkon Shield that she had—she woke up in a *pool* of blood—in her bed—and she went to the doctor and he said, "Oh, you'll have some extra bleeding with the Dalkon Shield" and advised her to keep it in. And every month she went through this, of having to use incredible amounts of—tampons and menstrual pads because she was bleeding so much. So, this went on for two years, and then—finally—what happened was the Dalkon Shield was embedded in her uterus, and they had to remove it, surgically.

A part of this story illustrates vividly the gender relations that informed women's experiences. The words, "She woke up in a pool of blood—in her bed—and she went to the doctor and he said, 'Oh, you'll have some extra bleeding with the Dalkon Shield,'" take us from the woman to a pool of blood in her bed, and then directly to the physician and his minimization of her experience. The bed is significantly situated between the image of the pool of blood and the image of the physician. Bed is one's safest place; a pool of blood in that bed is especially horrifying. Bed is also a place where contraceptives are needed. Yet we find no sexual partner here. The woman appears to be alone in the pool of blood in her bed. The only relationship that appears is that between the woman and her physician. For many women who use contraceptives that are not coitally related, the physician-patient relationship can become the most significant interaction in contraceptive use.

By the mid-1960s discussion began to appear in the medical literature about adverse effects reported by women using oral contraceptives. At the same time, articles began to appear discussing the psychological and psychiatric etiology of women's complaints about the pill. In September 1965 Drs. Richard Frank and Christopher Tietze published "Acceptance of an Oral Contraceptive Program in a Large Metropolitan Area" in the *American Journal of Obstetrics and Gynecology.* The protocol of the physicians' study betrayed their prejudices about the validity of women's complaints. They wrote, "Each patient received a two months' supply of pills at the first visit and was requested to return during the second month of Enovid medication. At this re-visit, it was ascertained that the patient still understood and followed the cyclic regimen and was given reassurances regarding any complaints she might experience." In this article reassurance was the only treatment prescribed for women who reported complaints about a potent drug that by that time was known to be associated with strokes, liver tumors, thromboembolism, and death.[13]

The same month an article appeared in *Good Housekeeping* communicating this professional attitude directly to women. The author wrote, "Dr. Pincus, research director of the Worcester Foundation for Experimental Biology, says that a study he made shows some side effects are caused by psychological responses, such as having heard that side effects are expected."[14] Dr. Pincus' attitude presented a paradox to women who kept informed about clinical experience with oral contraceptives. Some side effects were known to be, in some cases, signals of serious danger. An informed woman would want to report those symptoms promptly. The same symptoms, however—including headaches, dizziness, weakness, and "flu-like symptoms"—were also "known" to be "caused by psychological responses." An informed woman might not, therefore, report those symptoms.

In 1968 the *American Journal of Obstetrics and Gynecology* published "Psychiatric Reactions to Oral Contraceptives" by Dr. Francis J. Kane, Jr. Kane found that biological responses to the hormones in oral contraceptives could cause depressive illness:

> Alterations in biochemical amines, especially in the central nervous system, are seen as factors in onset and recovery from psychiatric illness, especially serious depressive illness. The experiments cited plus others indicating altered autonomic response with the use of gonadal hormones, seem to indicate that emotional disturbances should be, in a certain number of people using these hormones, an expectation rather than an occasion for surprise.[15]

Despite his findings, Kane was concerned with patients' fears about oral contraceptives. He cited the following study:

> Zell and Crisp categorized the fears with drug use: (1) Fears about bodily damage. While there can be some legitimate concern about such a possibility, these may also be a more superficial manifestation of resentment related to castration conflicts in women. Anything that might provoke physical change would be seen as a threat, especially if it were more likely to remind one more forcibly of their deprived female status. Such drugs might also diminish the possibility of using sexuality to manipulate a relationship with a man. (2) Fear of loss of control of sexual impulses and latent fantasies of prostitution. Such fears may account for some of the loss of sexual desire and capacity for orgasm seen in our sample.[16]

According to Kane, among the women in his study, "those who seem most 'conflicted' about their femininity seemed to experience the most symptomology." Apparently Kane's sample included many women who were "conflicted about their femininity." He acknowledged, "More than 50 percent of the population studied reported adverse effects, at least one quarter of whom felt badly enough to wish to stop the drug. . . . The evidence to date suggests an interaction of psychological and endocrine factors in the genesis of these disorders."[17] Kane did not explain how he concluded that reports of adverse effects were caused by conflicts about femininity, or why he did not consider an inverse relationship—that conflicts about femininity might be caused by the experience of adverse effects with contraceptive use.

Drs. Naomi Morris and J. Richard Udry published a study in August 1969 in which they found another physiological indication that oral contraceptives produced a depressive biologic effect. They did a comparison study of pedometer readings to measure the physical activity of pill users and nonusers, and found less activity in the group using oral contraceptives. They concluded that, "Since subjective fatigue and depression are widely recognized side effects of the pills, it seems reasonable to interpret the significant difference in pedometer readings as objective evidence of a depressant physiologic effect."[18]

Two months later an article appeared in the *American Journal of Obstetrics and Gynecology* claiming that side effects among users of oral contraceptives were produced by suggestion. The authors claimed, "Adverse publicity made many women anxious about the relationship of headaches and oral contraceptives. Yet most of them complained less when reassured that a serious problem would not arise from the symptoms. . . . Nowadays, after wider acceptance of these drugs [our colleagues] seldom see anyone with the complaint, whereas formerly they saw many treated women complaining of headaches."[19] By interpreting a decrease in *reports* of headaches as a decrease in *occurrence* of headaches, these physicians failed to recognize the possibility that women stopped talking about their headaches once they learned that their complaints would be met with reassurance and with suspicion. Many women might withhold complaints that are viewed by physicians as evidence of psychological instability.

When women had problems with intrauterine devices, physicians again offered reassurances in lieu of diagnosis and treatment. Those reassurances were widely reported in the popular media about the Dalkon Shield for six to ten years after the device was known to cause life-threatening problems. An FDA spokesman told reporters in 1974, "Doctors should consider removing the device . . . if it caused mental anguish in patients bothered by the reports of septic abortion and if it caused discomfort." The spokesman added, "On the basis of information currently available, we don't want to discourage women away from this means of contraception."[20]

A report six months later repeated the message to women: "The FDA has said that women currently using the Dalkon Shield without problems should continue using it." It was six *years* later that this message appeared: "Even if the women haven't suffered any problems related to the IUD . . . the device should be taken out because recent medical studies indicate a relationship between duration of IUD use and pelvic infection . . . [that] develops gradually . . . symptoms may not show up until an almond or walnut shaped mass develops in the pelvic area. By that time, the Fallopian tubes, ovaries or uterus may be so diseased that a complete hysterectomy would be necessary."[21]

Physicians' attitudes were responsible for some of the risks women interviewed for this project experienced. Gretchen used a Dalkon Shield after her physician failed to help her learn how to use a diaphragm. She was fortunate to be one of the women who may not have been injured by the device. Nancy was injured, and her treatment was delayed by her physician's attitude. When she had an acute attack of pelvic inflammatory disease, the first physician who examined her said that she had "just an irritation" from her IUD. Within a few days, an abscess was found on one of her ovaries.

Olivia was also injured. She was told that her complaints were the result of emotional problems. Olivia said, "I would bleed so heavily I would have to wear those pads like you wear after having a baby. I— almost didn't dare go out of the house unless I had one at the time. . . . I was really sick, cramps were unbelievable. . . . I was taking pain pills, but it was extremely painful, very uncomfortable, and it really knocked me out for eight to twelve days a month."

Olivia would sometimes experience sudden severe pain. She said, "If I was sitting and I would sneeze, I'd feel like somebody had ripped me apart inside." Her physician told her that the pain was psychosomatic. She said:

> I don't know if it had anything to do with when I finally went for surgery or not. I—was having a lot of pain, while I was having sex with my husband and they kept blaming it on *nerves*, because the year before the marriage broke up and—well, the marriage broke up around the same time the IUD was taken out. Just—so, but the year before we were having problems and they told me that I was emotional—having emotional problems and tension, and that was what was causing the pain.

Eventually physicians found objective evidence that Olivia's pain was physical—not emotional—in origin:

> But then when they did operate they—the doctor actually *apologized* because my uterus was—so malformed, misshapen they were going to remove it—it was on my right side—and they—first he tried to say I had a tipped uterus. And then finally when he opened—I didn't have a little band-aid surgery, he cut me wide across—and the uterus was here [Olivia positioned her hands over the right side of her lower abdomen] and he—formed it and put it back—hung it back up. Because he felt a girl at twenty-two should still have her periods. . . . So he did apologize and say that he had *really* been wrong. And then—that IUD was still *in,* and then I guess it was the next time I had my period he removed it.

Olivia said that it hurt when they removed her Dalkon Shield. "It was worse coming out . . . it was starting to—work its way into the wall. It had started to attach." Olivia later had abdominal surgery again, this time to remove adhesions from her bladder. She said she didn't know whether the problems with her bladder had been caused by the Dalkon Shield or by the surgery to repair her uterus.

While the physician-patient relationship is gender influenced, it is also sexually relevant for many women. Mary said that she was beginning to look for female doctors as much as possible, but she didn't want to switch to a female gynecologist. She explained, "Over the years, having the medical problems that I've had, I've tried to develop that type of medical—network—where people who are my doctors are also my friends. . . . I don't think you necessarily need a father figure. I think you just need someone you feel you can trust, and you can call him up and not have him say, 'Oh, you foolish woman.' " Mary liked her gynecologist, but not his partner. After relating some bad experiences she had with the partner, she said, "I started looking for female doctors as much as possible." But she was ambivalent about this. She said, "If you're going to expose yourself, you're going to expose yourself to a *man,* not to a woman. In your everyday sexual life and what-have-you, you're exposing those parts to a man, never to a woman."

The necessity of "exposing" herself to a man may have influenced Mary's delay in having her Dalkon Shield removed. Mary said that she put off having the device removed because her "life was very busy." She said she couldn't "think of any other reason that would have made me hesitate." I offered, "You said the insertion was painful," and Mary answered, "Oh, do you mean would I possibly have hesitated because of discomfort? I don't think so, I think I'm pretty logical about that stuff, you know, what has to be done has to be done, and you know, if it's going to hurt, so what? That too shall pass."

I then asked Mary what the insertion process had been like, and she said:

> I was surprised at how painful it was. I wouldn't say that it was excruciating, but I was *just* very surprised. The other thing I didn't like was that with the insertion or removal it's—at the time of your period, which I find very—difficult to—expose yourself psychologically at that time. I think you tend to be more emotional—I know I am—I tend to be—more fragile—more prone to upset or crying or—angry—or everything is—bigger. Yeah, that aspect I did not like, and I still would find that objectionable.

I asked Mary, "Does that have anything to do with being examined while you're menstruating?" and she answered:

> Oh, sure, sure. Half the time you don't really feel particularly—pleasant anyway—physically. You know, I think that aesthetically most people don't engage in sexual relations at that time. It is a time when you're discarding *waste.* So—previous to that—it's just not a pleasant time, you know. It's not a time when you would certainly choose. It's a time when you feel—most

vulnerable. You know, I've always—with my *medical* history doctors have always been *routine* for me, so, I'm not one to say, "Well, I don't want to go to the doctor," or, you know—I ask for my flu shot every year. I know friends of mine who just medically don't handle things. The idea of *blood* being drawn out of them—terrifies them. But I'm so used to—invasion, if you will—that that doesn't bother me much at all. Yet at that point the insertion during my period did bother me. I really don't think that's—*pleasant*.

The fact that removal of the Dalkon Shield would also occur while she was menstruating might help to explain why this health-conscious woman found that her life was so very busy that she risked losing it by waiting too long to have the device removed.

Olivia's comments about the pain of IUD insertion were preceded by her acknowledgment that she had been embarrassed. Asked, "Do you remember the process—when he actually inserted it, what that was like for you?" Olivia answered, "Well, other than being embarrassed—in that position—I remember—that you had to have your period so that you'd be—open wider. And it was—painful."

Nina's description of the IUD insertion identified her sense of having been invaded against her will. She said, "It was uncomfortable. I don't like the way they open up the uterus when the uterus isn't—wanting to be opened up."

It was evident in the interviews that normal gender and sexual relationships were reflected in the relationship between female patients and their male gynecologists. The norm extended to cover the full range of potential relationships between men and women. Gretchen's experience with her gynecologist was one of paternalism, in which Gretchen was "scolded [and] yelled at" when she didn't insert the diaphragm correctly. She said the physician wouldn't let her leave until she did what he told her to do. She described that experience as humiliating.

Melissa described an experience with a physician that was suggestive of rape:

I went back for a checkup and the doctor said I had an erosion that was probably caused from the Dalkon Shield and that I should have it cauterized. I was on Medicaid at the time, and . . . which I think was related to what happened without my, without my knowledge—without my permission. Anyway, he immediately stuck the machine in me and turned—stuck this thing in me and turned on this machine that made this big noise and I said, "What are you doing?" and he said, "I'm—this is cryosurgery." And I didn't know what cryosurgery was. All I—all I heard was the word "surgery." It was a pretty horrible experience—because, because he hadn't explained—why he was doing it or, I was given no choice about it. It was a pretty awful experience—traumatic—and I'm not convinced that was, that cryosurgery had to be done. Maybe, maybe it would have healed on its own. The way it was handled was horrible because I—I wasn't consulted, I didn't know what was happening, I thought he was cutting off my cervix for all I knew because I was just pretty—even though I had started learning about my body, I certainly didn't know what cryosurgery was—and I just really didn't *know*—too much about it. *Physically* what happened was I felt I was being—what they do is they use—I think it's carbon dioxide. It's—very cold—very—I don't know—but anyway, I felt like I was being blown up like a balloon, which you do actually absorb the carbon dioxide. When the procedure was *over*, when they took the thing *off*, I started to get up from the table because I was really angry and upset, and the nurse came and—whammed her hand against my chest—and shoved me back down on the table and said, "You can't get up." Neither of them told me why I can't get up; I was like—*captured* there, and I was *crying*. I finally got it together to say, "*Why* can't I get up?" and they said, "Because of the carbon dioxide, it's changed—it's chemically changed something in your body, and if you get up, you'll faint." I realized I really might faint, because I'd started to feel dizzy—they were right about that, but they—the way they did it was—terrible.

For some of the women interviewed, experience with contraceptive injuries sharpened their identification with the shared concerns of women. Anna considered herself an emancipated woman at the time that she purchased her Dalkon Shield. Her experience with that device transformed her understanding of the meaning of emancipation and the meaning of women's oppression:

It was like my whole being had been *scrambled*. Like I'd been put in a blender. And I came out—I really didn't know what I *was*. You know, I just—I didn't know—I didn't know anything—about myself really—until this happened. I didn't know really what my *values* were. I mean obviously I *did*. I was a functioning—person. But—at the *level* that this—forced me—to make choices, and, priorities. I was—totally shocked. I mean partly because of—because of the evolution of my feminism, and—and the fact that I was always a very—sort of male-oriented feminist—it was *hard* for me to work in the—the—the traditional, the traditional *female* aspects of what I was going through. It was very, very hard for me. Because I had never thought of myself in those terms. I mean to have—all of, a lot of, my Marxist—feminist—friends that I had been working with politically and intellectually for a *year* were not all that—sympathetic. Whereas people that I had *nothing* in common with—were *unbelievably* sympathetic. And that totally threw me. Because I ended up turning for support to people that—I had—very little in *common* with—which was bizarre—but wonderful. I mean it totally transformed my relationship with my family, with women in my family, absolutely.

Megan, now an activist working in AIDS education, said that her experience with the Dalkon Shield made her a feminist. She explained, "It was really my experience with the Dalkon Shield that pissed me off enough, you know, to really start getting involved in women's organizations and to know more, and to become more active. . . . Thanks to A. H. Robins, I became a feminist." Megan was twenty-two years old when she purchased her Dalkon Shield. She was married and had never had a child. After becoming pregnant with the shield in place, Megan suffered a miscarriage. She recalled:

> I had the Dalkon Shield put in—I think it was about 1973—because I had heard great things about IUDs. I would have been twenty-two. After being on the pill as my only means of contraception, at that point, the idea of using a diaphragm or something that you had to deal with at the moment—was like, "No!"—you wanted the spontaneity, and all that.
>
> At that point in time I think people were concerned about the effects of the pill. And this seemed to offer, in fact, even more spontaneity in that one didn't have to do anything with it. At the time it was really being touted as the perfect method of contraception, with high efficacy rates, and one needed to do nothing to have it. I think I had heard that there was a possibility that it might cause severe cramping, and that if your body didn't adjust to it, then it wasn't a method you should use. But I had it about three years without it causing any problems.
>
> Then, in 1976, I had a miscarriage. Two months earlier I had actually called Planned Parenthood, because there was starting to be stuff about the Dalkon Shield at the time. And I said, "I've got the Dalkon Shield, and I kind of wonder if I should have it taken out." I was still real hooked on IUDs, and wanted to get another kind put in. And their response was, "Well, how long have you had it?" and I said "About three years." And they said, "Well, if you've had it that long and your body hasn't rejected it, chances are you're O.K. with it. It's all right for you. And if we took that one out and put another

kind in, that might be more traumatic for your body than just leaving the Shield in." So that made a certain amount of sense to me, and I left it in.

My husband and I were trying to get our marriage back together at the time, and I realized I was pregnant—with the shield in place—and really couldn't decide what I was going to do. My husband was, to say the least, quite unhappy. He tried to be decent about it, to his credit, but he was just not really prepared to face the prospect of us getting our marriage back together and of me being pregnant. He really wanted me to get an abortion, and I was very ambivalent. I went in and talked to some people in a women's clinic, and they were really wonderful. I even went so far as to make an appointment for an abortion. I knew it was not very good to get pregnant with the shield anyway— this is not your best way to start out a pregnancy. And clearly it was unintended. But I still felt very ambivalent about the abortion, and I called a friend of mine and told her the whole situation. She said to me, "Well, what do *you* want to do?" And I said to her, "I want to have the baby." And she said, "Well, do it!" It was just her asking me that simple flat-out question, "What did I want?" instead of "What does this guy you're married to want?" or "What are you supposed to do?" And she said, "You can come back here and live with us." And I decided that was what I was going to do. My husband was—not delighted—and it was clear that this was kind of the last nail in the marital coffin.

I found out that if I had the Dalkon Shield removed and tried to continue the pregnancy, I would have a 25 percent chance of having a miscarriage. If I left it in, I had a 75 percent chance of having a septic abortion. And I thought that the latter one didn't sound so hot. So I went to the doctor, and he removed the shield. Everything seemed cool for a couple of days, and then I started bleeding, and I spent a week in bed, making great promises to things up there in the sky, "Oh, well, if you'll let me be O.K., I'll be good for the rest of my life."

But I wound up in the hospital, finishing off this miscarriage. We walked in, and told the nurse what was happening, and she calls out, "Get her out of here. I don't want her bleeding all over the floor!" So—I spent a couple of days in the hospital from that. I remember lying on the gurney in the emergency room and watching this big clock on the wall. I think I was the least of their concerns that night, you know, "She wasn't going to *die*" or anything. And there was *lots* of blood on the floor and everything, all around. And whoever the doctor was—it wasn't my doctor there in the emergency room at the time— but I remember the doctor was coming up and was touching me very softly on the arm and was saying, "I think you lost your baby."

Megan changed her mind about the importance of convenience in selecting a method of contraception after she used the Dalkon Shield:

Oral contraceptives, IUDs—not that they're not *convenient* for women—they are convenient, but they're also—at worst—deadly. And they're not worth it to me, any more. . . . I think there are a lot of advantages to a diaphragm. The one being that it's been around—for a long time, and—the side effects are—pretty nil. I mean, there are—can be some for certain women. Some women don't adapt to them well—have more—more of a tendency toward urinary infection, or whatever. But that's—that's much more manageable than *PID,* you know—hysterectomy, perforated uterus—I've yet to hear of somebody finding a diaphragm lodged in somebody's intestines. And I think, too, with the diaphragm you have to learn something about your anatomy, your own body. You have—it becomes a *shared* responsibility. You can *teach* your partner—how to put it in. And if—you know—if you're dealing with a partner who [Megan made a face, as if to portray disgust in the partner]—then you kick him out of bed; "Oh, that's gross!" "Well, not as gross as your attitude, out!" And I don't think it's so bad to stop and say, well here's what we've got to do. We've got to remember, you know, as much *fun* as sex is, and as lovely and wonderful, that—you can—create pregnancy. You can get pregnant from sex. And I don't think that's such a bad thing for folks to remember.

Megan said that she decided, "There was going to be no more of this, 'Oh, pardon me dear,' and then going off to put it in and then coming back. Instead it's, 'I'm putting it in. I'm here. If you don't like it, go *sleep* somewhere else!' There's none of this, 'Let's pretend we're Ozzie and Harriet from the fifties.' Because I was so angry—I was just so angry."

Her experience with the Dalkon Shield made Megan cynical about technological innovations for contraception. She said, "Even if someone said tomorrow, 'Eureka! We've found the perfect method of contraception,' I'd say, 'Well, I'm thirty-seven now, you come and you let me know when I'm seventy how good it's been in the last thirty-odd years—and maybe *then* I'll try it. . . .'"

Tension between the desire to control procreative power responsibly and the ultimate wish to maintain it was consistently expressed by the women I interviewed. For some of them, an inadvertent pregnancy would have interrupted career plans; for others, it would present a financial burden. In some cases, an inadvertent pregnancy would publicize the breaking of sexual mores by presenting evidence of sexual involvement;

in others, it would have brought recriminations that the woman had failed to use her contraceptive correctly. Each of these social factors contributed to an urgent attempt by women to assure that the contraceptives they used were effective. Safety—freedom from bodily harm— often became a secondary consideration.

Women expressed ambivalence about men's role in contraceptive use. The desire for men to use contraception and for new methods to be made available to men was often expressed. But many women wanted to control their own fertility, and did not want to turn responsibility over to men. Some said they did not trust men with that responsibility. Others worried about the male ego. Still others worried about the physical safety of methods designed for men. Some women were particularly concerned that the fertility and sexual response of men should be protected. Those concerns were also expressed in the medical and family planning literature.

The 1960s was identified as a time when revolutionary new developments in birth control promised a "sexual revolution" in which the responsibility of procreative control could be forever separated from coitus. Many women said that this convenience had been a factor in their choice of contraceptive method. Experts hailed coitally unrelated birth control as the answer to "man's [sic] ancient dream" of achieving "gay abandon" in sexual expression.

For women, no such "gay abandon" materialized. The removal of the mechanics of birth control from the coital moment changed the social relationships of sexuality for women. Technologically sophisticated methods of contraception increased the involvement of physicians in the intimate—and embarrassing—necessities of procreative control for many women. The attitudes of physicians, and the feelings of women about their bodies, their bodily functions, and their sexuality, influenced the treatment women received when they were injured. It also influenced their choice of birth control method and their success in learning to use traditional methods. Because most physicians were men, problems related to gender dichotomy and gender oppression were salient features in two relationships related to contraceptive use: the relationship between women and their coital partners, and the relationship between women and their physicians.

Injury from contraceptive use changed some women's minds about the advantages of separating the responsibilities of procreative control from the time and place of coitus. The recognition of responsibility by both partners for the consequences of sexual involvement was viewed as more liberating to women than the separation of that responsibility had been. The separation of responsibility from coitus turned out to have been no more than an extension of the division of labor by sex to the sexual relationship itself.

5   New Products, Old Problems

In the three decades since the initial introduction of oral contraceptives, health problems associated with their use have brought a series of changes in the manufacture, regulation, and use of contraceptive products. In the 1970s, lower-dosage pills were developed in the hope that milder doses would cause fewer and less severe side effects. The U.S. Food and Drug Administration decided to require package inserts that would inform women of some of the health risks known to be associated with oral contraceptive use. Health and family planning professionals sought alternative methods that would not sacrifice the effectiveness of the pills. Many women changed their method of contraception, often switching to intrauterine devices. Pharmaceutical companies looked forward to an expanding market for new products, particularly IUDs. Competition became intense among scientists and businessmen to develop and patent the perfect contraceptive. Physicians took an increasing interest in the promising business of contraceptive innovation.

Another set of changes followed in the wake of the Dalkon Shield case. The FDA mandated stricter guidelines for the testing of contraceptive products. Many women have considered barrier methods, hoping to avoid the potential hazards of both pills and intrauterine devices. Family planning groups have pushed for the development of new, highly use-effective methods that will be more acceptable to women. Proponents of population control have increased their research and development activities as pharmaceutical companies have cut back on the development of new products. All but one manufacturer of IUDs ceased marketing the devices in the United States several years ago; recently new IUDs have been introduced here again. The marketing of IUDs has never stopped worldwide. New products have features reminiscent of IUDs: they require little user control; they cannot be used without being introduced into the body by health care professionals; their mode of action is not completely understood; their potential hazards are the subject of heated debate; and they provide a long-term contraceptive effect. While proponents of population control have struggled to secure FDA approval of these products, women's health advocates have fought to prevent the usurpation by the state and by professionals of women's power to exercise procreative choice.

As the search for a perfect method of contraception continues, the motivations and values of the various interest groups involved in that search remain fundamentally unchanged. But the rhetoric of population control has changed. In 1978, a hearing was held before the U.S. House of Representatives to discuss the injectable contraceptive called Depo-Provera. The drug had been used in Third World countries for more than a decade, but the FDA had not approved its use in the United States for the purpose of fertility regulation. The drug had been used in the United States on a limited basis without FDA approval, and had been tested for eleven years at a metropolitan hospital in Atlanta, primarily on poor black women. Use of the drug had been associated with a number of complications, including breast cancer, stroke, amenorrhea, headaches, weight gain, permanent infertility, loss of libido, and congenital problems in fetuses, including clitoral hypertrophy, cardiac defects, and limb reduction.[1]

As in government investigations of the pill and IUDs, debate about the regulation of Depo-Provera centered around the issue of risk/benefit assessment. On one side stood those who claimed that the health risks were too great to justify the approval of the drug; on the other side, those who argued that the drug's benefits outweighed any hazards associated with its use. Supporters of Depo-Provera approval accused opponents of western elitism and an antifeminist bias. Proclaiming that they were the true defenders of the health of women and children, supporters claimed that for some women pregnancy was more hazardous than Depo-Provera.

The following remarks were typical of those supporting FDA approval of Depo-Provera:

> When you have such high maternal and infant mortality in the developing world, how can you retreat to your academic chambers and debate whether the risk of X, Y, or Z is point aught something to point aught something else,

when we are talking about the immediate life-threatening risk of pregnancy? I still have the feeling that you are approaching this whole thing on a Western model that is quite inappropriate to the desperate urgency and need in the developing world. . . . Depo-Provera has been subjected to over six million women-years of use and monitoring. It is safe, it is efficient, it is convenient. We ask in the name of suffering women of the less developed countries, the women condemned to death and disease from repeated childbearing and its related problems, that the ban be lifted and DMPA be permitted for general use.[2]

One speaker attacked feminist health activists directly:

I'd just like to remind the Chairman that we're not here today because of Depo-Provera itself, but because of the human suffering that the lack of it has caused and will cause. I got into this issue because of that suffering. I had answered one too many letters from women in the developing world who want this drug. The fact that U.S. feminists have come forth and maligned this drug has resulted in its denial to a lot of women, and has caused a tremendous amount of human suffering.[3]

Representatives of the International Planned Parenthood Federation were among the supporters of FDA approval of the drug. While the U.S. Food and Drug Administration had no jurisdiction over the use of products in other countries, the claim was made that "without any kind of approval in this country, the drug will continue to be 'politically suspect' and, as a result, won't be made as widely available." Population control efforts abroad could be expanded through the use of Depo-Provera once it was approved by the FDA, it was argued, because "the political reality is that U.S. decisions do carry great weight overseas."[4]

Feminist critics of Depo-Provera pointed out that the drug was not the only alternative to pregnancy for women, and that women in developing countries had access to safer methods of contraception. Asked to respond to that criticism, one spokesman for Depo-Provera said:

No woman anywhere is faced with the choice of Depo-Provera or no contraception. Indigenous and traditional contraceptives—abstinence, withdrawal, prolonged lactation, various forms of rhythm technique, the use of leaves, gums, mud as barriers—these are contraceptives available everywhere. Further, induced abortion—legal or otherwise—is used almost everywhere to control unwanted fertility. For a highly motivated couple, some of these, especially abstinence and withdrawal, are certainly safe and effective contraceptives. Why then Depo-Provera? Because many couples are willing to accept the health risks and the short-term side effects of Depo-Provera because of the convenience it offers, the sexual freedom it allows, the practical and emotional difficulties of other forms of contraception it avoids, all this coupled with very high effectiveness that does not require extremely high—perhaps unrealistically high—motivation by the user.[5]

As with intrauterine devices, it was the use-effectiveness of Depo-Provera that prompted its promotion by members of the international population control community. Its use-effectiveness was cited as a benefit that would apply to some populations of women in the United States, as well as to women in developing countries:

> Even among the vast population of the United States, you can find sub-groups of people who have the same problems as people in the developing world. . . . I think that if the FDA were to turn its attention to the needs of some of the sub-groups within the United States, we would not be faced with the situation in which we can be accused of having a dual standard of medical practice and drug regulation around the world. If you look hard enough in the United States, I think you can find the same type of population—as I say—it might not be very large—as one finds in the north of Thailand.[6]

The size and composition of the potential U.S. market for Depo-Provera was considered by several witnesses. Asked, "Could you define the sub-groups within the U.S.A. population where the risk-benefit ratio of contraceptive use differs from the general population?" Dr. Malcolm Potts answered, "Minority populations in the U.S.A. suffer a higher mortality than white Americans. For pooled data, the differential is approximately threefold and has persisted over recent years and during an interval when maternal mortality has declined." Dr. H. K. Toppozada answered the same question by identifying six groups of women for whom he thought the benefits of Depo-Provera would outweigh the risks. Those women included: "Those who have completed their families or those with a minimum of at least three children; cases who are intolerant to or who have a contraindication to the use of estrogens or IUDs; subjects who are not bothered by cycle disturbances or prolonged amenorrhea; those who are liable to forget or get mixed up about the daily intake of oral contraceptives; women living in rural areas; and lactating women." Dr. E. M. Coutinho offered his list of potential users: "Mental cases. Women with endometrial hyperplasia who cannot take estrogenic contraceptives and should not wear IUDs. Undernourished women for whom amenorrhea may be beneficial. Women who do not tolerate oral estrogens and who refuse IUDs." Another physician, Dr. R. A. Hatcher, felt that Depo-Provera "would probably be a superb drug for many teenagers." Later in Dr. Hatcher's testimony he discussed a problem peculiar to teenagers using the drug. He said, "There's some evidence with oral contraceptives that those most susceptible to post-pill amenorrhea are very, very young teenagers, and I imagine the same might be demonstrated with Depo-Provera. I imagine it would be a low level of risk, however."[7] Dr. Hatcher named ten additional groups of women who were, "considered by us, by the clinicians working with me, to be the clinical settings where we would be most likely to use Depo-Provera":

> Women who want no more children, but who do not want a sterilization procedure performed; women who want a safe, effective method of birth control for a short period of time prior to sterilization; women over 30 years old; women who are mentally retarded; women receiving rubella vaccine who must be protected against pregnancy for three months; women with sickle cell disease; women who have experienced unplanned pregnancies or medical complications with other methods, or who refuse to use other methods; women at particularly high risk of developing cardiovascular complications from estrogen-containing birth control pills; women who have developed certain estrogen or estrogen-related side effects from combined oral contraceptives, such as headaches, high blood pressure, leg pain or chloasma; and women who are being evaluated for suspicious pap smears, so that they do not become pregnant during the period of evaluation.[8]

Dr. T. B. Hubbard was among the witnesses who supported the approval of Depo-Provera use. He considered Depo-Provera an appropriate solution to both social and personal problems. He said, "The morbidity and mortality, as well as the social pathology associated with unwanted pregnancies and unwanted children, far outweigh the demonstrated or even the extreme theoretical risks of using either Depo-Provera or the oral contraceptives."[9]

Depo-Provera exceeds even the intrauterine devices in its ability to displace control of procreative power from the woman to the physician. Once injected into the bloodstream, a dose of Depo-Provera cannot be withdrawn by anyone. One shot of Depo-Provera can have a contraceptive effect that lasts for many months—even years—depending on the strength of the dosage. In some women, sterility becomes permanent. No woman receiving a shot of Depo-Provera can be certain how large a dose she is being given. No woman can change her mind and decide to stop using the drug, either because she cannot tolerate the side effects or because she wants to become pregnant. The drug has to wear off before fertility can recur. Once fertility does return, if it ever does, it is not clear how soon a woman can safely become pregnant without damage to the fetus. Any woman who becomes gravely ill from the drug must consult a physician in the hope of having other drugs administered to counteract the effects of Depo-Provera. The effects of combining drugs is not known. Once Depo-Provera is injected into her bloodstream, a woman loses all control over its effect on her body, her fertility, and her life. Yet it is that very loss of control by the woman that makes Depo-Provera an almost perfect method of birth control, according to its supporters.

The Depo-Provera battle is not over. The National Women's Health Network reports that it is still engaged in a desperate effort to keep the drug from being approved by the FDA, and, in an equally desperate effort, to inform women who are being exposed to the drug in the United States and around the world that it is a dangerous and potentially lethal drug.[10]

Meanwhile, women in the United States still, at the discretion of their health care providers, get Depo-Provera for contraceptive use. Physicians do not have to have permission from the FDA to prescribe the drug. The drug is unapproved for contraceptive use, but it is not banned. Some physicians, however, refuse to administer a drug that has not been approved, fearing litigation in case of injury. No one knows how many women have actually used Depo-Provera. As with oral contraceptives, the long-term systemic effects, which could be passed on through generations of progeny, will not be known during this century.

Depo-Provera is no longer the only injectable contraceptive available. In 1987 *Population Reports* named four brands that were being marketed around the world. Two had been developed by corporations—Depo-Provera by Upjohn and Net-En by Schering; the World Health Organization's Human Reproduction Project had developed the other two. All the injectables contain progestin, a sex hormone. Although estrogen is sometimes prescribed along with these products to relieve side effects, the fact that they do not contain estrogen is counted as a major advantage and featured in their promotion.

Two other progestin products are being used by women in many countries. Silastic (a type of plastic) rods filled with progestin are implanted under the skin of the upper arm; their contraceptive effect lasts five years. The rods must be implanted and removed by health care professionals. While the contraceptive effect supposedly ends immediately when the rods are withdrawn, this claim is controversial. The side effects of the implants are the same as for the injectable progestins, and the long-term effects on women and their children are equally unpredictable. The same drug is available on a more limited basis in vaginal rings. The rings are less desirable to professionals who value little user control. The local and systemic effects of the rings are as controversial as the effects of injectables and implantables. In 1983 Johns Hopkins' Population Information Program reported that progestin products were being used by hundreds of thousands of women in more than one hundred countries. Recently the implants were approved for marketing in the United States despite the long fight of women's health advocates to block that approval.[11]

Intrauterine devices remain a popular method among international family planners. In 1986 the most widely used IUDs in the United States were withdrawn from the domestic market in response to the effects of litigation. The manufacturer's insurance company had refused to renew the liability policy for Searle, who made the Copper 7 and the Tatum T devices. The "explosion of lawsuits—and the cost of insuring against them"—was blamed for the "limiting" of women's choices. Only one IUD remained available in the United States, and that one was many times more expensive than earlier models. Research and testing of IUDs by private foundations went on in this country. Dissemination of IUDs to women in other countries continued. In 1987 the Population Information Program found a company willing to manufacture and market a "new generation" IUD in the United States.[12]

The new device, TCu-380A, also called Para-Gard, is sold by the GynoPharma Pharmaceutical Company of New Jersey. *Population Reports* announced this development in March 1988 and explained the "advantages" the device would have for family planning programs in other parts of the world. The report stated, "The U.S. situation may have been misunderstood. For example, in an informal 1986 survey, nine of 29 African planning directors said that they thought most IUDs were no longer sold in the U.S. because they were declared unsafe. . . . The directors did not realize that the manufacturers' decisions were primarily financial. Introduction of the TCu-380A in the U.S. should help to correct these misunderstandings."[13]

The idea that withdrawal of IUDs from the U.S. market was simply a business decision is widespread. It is argued that court decisions favoring plaintiffs in the Dalkon Shield case set a precedent that encouraged other IUD users to file suits against manufacturers. While some reports are sympathetic to all manufacturers—including A. H. Robins—others acknowledge the legitimacy of claims in the Dalkon Shield case but challenge the claims made against other intrauterine devices. According to that argument, fear of litigation and the withdrawal of liability coverage by insurance companies have created a crisis for manufacturers. That litigation is brought against manufacturers as a result of devastating injuries goes unrecognized or unacknowledged.

Population Reports is correct, of course, in asserting that business considerations did finally prompt corporations to stop selling IUDs in the United States. Reports of injuries and deaths of women, which came years before the devices were withdrawn, never had that effect. It took litigation—successful litigation—by injured women and the survivors of women who died to force the temporary removal of IUDs from the market.

The March 1988 issue of *Population Reports* made it clear that business considerations will continue to prevail over women's safety. This message was printed in a boxed commentary entitled, "What's in a Name?"

> GynoPharma, the company that will market the TCu-380A in the U.S., used focus-group discussions (small group discussions with a trained interviewer) and surveys to decide on the name Para-Gard for the TCu-380A. Market research found that, to potential users, the name Para-Gard suggests a modern and effective IUD. GynoPharma favors the name because "Para" suggests to doctors an IUD for parous women. Their research suggests that women usually accept their doctor's recommendation for an IUD. . . . Social marketing programs in many countries have given attention to naming contraceptives that are purchased directly by consumers. Names chosen for oral contraceptives—such as Gulaf, meaning rose, in Nepal and Maya, meaning affection, in Bangladesh—suggest femininity and caring. Names chosen for condoms, such as Panther in various countries, and Raja, meaning king in Bangladesh, suggest strength and masculinity. . . . In contrast, little effort has been given to finding IUD names that appeal to users. Although a good name cannot substitute for a good IUD, an appealing name coupled with a catchy logo and attractive packaging could help to promote a positive image of IUDs and heighten interest among potential users.[14]

Part of the sales pitch for the IUDs that are available now is that they do not have the Dalkon Shield's design flaws. The cause of complications from that device has been reduced in the popular imagination to a matter of design. No attention is given to the evidence that *all* IUDs have been associated with foreign body reactions that predispose tissue to infection.

No attention has been given, either, to the evidence that infectious organisms responsible for IUD infections are many, varied, and can come from a woman's own body. The claim is made that the monogamous woman need not fear IUD infection, which is erroneously said to be caused exclusively by sexual transmission of disease. IUDs are recommended primarily for women who have already had children. This rationale rests on the premise that every woman *should* have one child, and that fertility can thereafter be compromised. There is nothing anatomical about a parous woman to suggest that IUD use is not hazardous for her. The value of a woman's fertility still corresponds with her social worth, as decided by professionals concerned with population control. The health and the lives of millions of women remain expendable in the interest of maintaining "civilization as we know it."

In March 1988 *Ms.* magazine published "A Failed Revolution" by Ellen Sweet. The caption under the headline read, "We expected the perfect contraceptive by now, but our choices are more limited than ever before. . . . Ellen Sweet's investigation found that bottom-line pressure and liability risks have caused the major drug companies to give up the search." The author wrote, "The expectation of no-hassle, highly effective birth control dates from the marketing of the pill in 1960, followed a few years later by the IUD. Now, we have an improved, lower dosage, safer Pill; and the sponge has been added to the older forms of birth control—the diaphragm, condom, spermicides, rhythm method, and sterilization. But we have lost most IUDs."[15]

Writing about the new Para-Gard, Sweet said, "One improvement in design is a single filament polyethylene string, which is less likely to attract bacteria than the multifilament tail that experts in the Dalkon Shield trial cited as a probable source of PID and other infections." No other source of PID is identified in this article, although the author acknowledged that the IUD "is still advised for women over 25, who do not want to have children and who are in a stable relationship."[16]

Citing litigation as the cause of roadblocks preventing contraceptive innovation, Sweet listed the new methods she found "most intriguing." Among them were injectable and implantable progestins, vaginal rings, silicone plugs to block oviducts, a chemical modification of a brain hormone that suppresses ova or sperm production, and several surgical and chemical products for men, including Gossypol.[17] Sweet expressed some ambivalence about the more cautious attitude of the FDA in recent years:

> The FDA's rigorous requirements for approval of drugs intended for healthy people protect women from some of the worst potential health problems. Before the dangers of the Dalkon Shield became apparent, the FDA regulated

medications such as the Pill, but there were no rules governing contraceptive devices. Women's health groups considered the introduction of such requirements as a victory, yet now a relatively simple product, the cervical cap, had to undergo extensive animal testing before it was allowed to enter clinical trials here.[18]

According to Doris Haire, Chair of the Committee on Health Law and Regulation of the National Women's Health Network, "The power and the inclination of the FDA to protect women is still very limited. The FDA still defines 'safe' as a relative term, based on . . . what the FDA considers to be the acceptable potential risks and benefits of the particular drug." The FDA still relies on manufacturers to submit data on safety prior to a drug's approval. Once a drug is marketed, the FDA relies on manufacturers and physicians—who have vested interests in avoiding liability for injury—to report adverse reactions. Data on safety are protected as trade secrets by the FDA and are not available to the public. Haire wrote, "FDA approval of a drug as safe does not automatically mean that the drug has been subjected to properly controlled scientific evaluation and follow-up of individuals exposed to the direct and indirect effects of the drug. The Director of the FDA's Bureau of Drugs has confirmed in writing that the FDA does not guarantee the safety of any drug—not even those which the FDA has officially approved as safe."[19]

The withdrawal or withholding of contraceptive products from the market does limit women's choices. When the products kept from women are dangerous, however, that limitation scarcely curtails benefits. To use a potentially dangerous method of contraception is to exchange one set of risks for another. The risk of pregnancy is exchanged for the risk of contraceptive injury; the risks of injury from one product are exchanged for the risks of injury by another. Promoters of "new-generation" products have historically made the most of that exchange of risks, selling one product as free of the risks found in some previously devastating product. The entire risk-exchange process stands as an alternative to one other risk that we stubbornly avoid confronting: the risk of having openly to challenge the existing social and cultural relationships that define the parameters of procreative choice in the first place.

6 Trading Risks

In the case of the Dalkon Shield, many risks derived from the structure of the health care system. As an integral part of a capitalist economic system that is global in its reach, the U.S. health care system reflects and reinforces normal capitalist social relationships. Decisions made by "experts" about the Dalkon Shield often had more to do with the health of financial interests than they did with the health of individual women. The device was designed and tested by a man who made a substantial profit from its sale. As a physician, that man was in a position of cultural authority that made the "scientific" promotion of his product credible to the profession and to the consumer. After its inventor sold the Dalkon Shield to the A. H. Robins Corporation he was hired as a consultant for the corporation. Again, his cultural authority as a physician was used to sell the product. His book about intrauterine devices, written as if it were an authoritative and objective study of IUDs, was used as propaganda in an international advertising campaign for the sale of Dalkon Shields.

The data that went to the Food and Drug Administration to establish the safety of the Dalkon Shield was supplied by the A. H. Robins Corporation. The FDA used a risk/benefit analysis to decide that the device was safe to market. It took nearly twenty years from the first known insertion of a Dalkon Shield into a woman's body for a public advertising campaign to be launched warning women that they should have the devices removed. The injuries caused by the device had been a matter of public record for at least 15 years before the warning came. The campaign to have Dalkon Shields removed from the bodies of women came as a response to litigation, not as a response to mutilation and death. It was confined to the United States, where the bulk of litigation was pending. No effort was ever made by the corporation to inform women in the eighty other countries where the Dalkon Shield was marketed that the device could maim and kill.

Little about the Dalkon Shield case was unusual. It is not unusual for scientists working on innovations in health care to be interested in profiting from their discoveries. In a capitalist system, physicians are businesspersons who profit from their research and their professional practices. It is not unusual for physicians to work as consultants for corporations, providing authoritative backing for the sale of the corporations' products.

The FDA routinely relies on manufacturers to supply the data on which it bases regulatory decisions. Those decisions routinely involve the value judgments inherent in a risk/benefit analysis and a subjective definition of safety. Decisions made by the FDA routinely reflect economic and political interests. The risk/benefit analysis of the FDA about the safety of contraceptive products is routinely expressed in the language of population control politics, which is the parlance of economic dominance and political imperialism. Population control enthusiasts fear revolution from populations who have been denied access to the wealth generated by world capitalism. Scarcity produced by the misappropriation of the planet's resources by a tiny percentage of the earth's inhabitants has been blamed on the size of the populations who produced but who have been denied that wealth. In the scientific risk/benefit analysis of contraceptive products social control is considered a benefit outweighing the substantial risks to women.

The information available to consumers about the Dalkon Shield came from the same health care system that produced the device. Its content was determined by the same economic and political interests and value judgments that influenced innovation, testing, manufacture, regulation, and distribution of the device. Hegemonic interests that declared the Dalkon Shield safe and a revolutionary product among new-generation IUDs continue to endanger all consumers in a capitalist economy. The Dalkon Shield is one of many products that have maimed and killed consumers.

The dumping of Dalkon Shields in the Third World after sales were stopped in the United States was not an unusual event, either. The dumping of dangerous pesticides, outdated drugs, and pajamas containing carcinogenic materials banned in the United States was exposed by Mark

Dowie and Barbara Ehrenreich in the same article in which they exposed the dumping of the Dalkon Shield in 1979.[1] Not only unsafe products, but unsafe manufacturing procedures have been exported to protect profits. The poisoning of the people of Bhopal by lethal gases and the poisoning of children in Mexico by carelessly discarded asbestos are two examples in a seemingly endless list of atrocities.

The targeting of poor women and women of color as subgroups for whom differential treatment is proposed was also not exceptional. Historically, both men and women have had sterilization procedures forced upon them when advantaged people decided that the disadvantaged should be denied procreation for the good of humanity. Imperialism has been rationalized on the premise that disadvantaged people are too ignorant or too lazy to control their own lives. New developments in contraceptive and reproductive technologies promise more weapons in the same war. By the turn of the century, poor men and men of color, particularly in the Third World, may well find themselves the targets of mass efforts that rival those that have been directed at women for more than thirty years. Already testing of contraceptives for men has been initiated in the Third World, just as the initial tests of pills, IUDs, injectables, and implantables were begun on Third World women.

Even among contraceptive products the Dalkon Shield was not unique. Oral contraceptives have a similar history. All IUDs have been associated with most of the same risks that women faced with the Dalkon Shield. The manufacture, testing, regulation, and distribution of all contraceptives takes place within the same social context. Newer methods carry social risks of global proportions as well as potential physical risks that could prove to be of equal or greater magnitude.

The method I used in this study made the attempt to answer my primary questions an arduous task. I studied the problem from the top down, from the ground up, and from the inside out. The study of the health care system, the political context, and the economic interests represented in this case constituted a top down approach. The study of women's narratives about their experiences with contraception represented a ground up approach. By beginning with open-ended questions designed to generate rather than test theory, I was also using an approach that forced me to work from inside the problem out toward a theoretical understanding.

Had I studied the problem only from the top down, considering social structure as the primary determinant of women's lives, I might have found the hierarchy of oppression I was looking for. I might have been able to make a case for seeing clear distinctions between women of different classes, races, and countries that correlated with the amount of oppression a given woman could be expected to have suffered. Professionals did target some populations of women for less careful treatment than they recommended for others. Less care could be taken in the dissemination of potentially dangerous contraceptives to poor and disadvantaged women, it was claimed, because those women—in the United States and especially in the Third World—needed use-effective methods more than middle-class white American women did. More cautious care was prescribed for privileged women both in the insertion of IUDs and in the treatment of complications.

Within the literature addressing the relationship of gender and sex to population control efforts, Betsy Hartmann's *Reproductive Rights and Wrongs: The Global Politics of Population Control and Contraceptive Choice* is the most recent and perhaps the most exhaustive study available. Hartmann views the sexual oppression of Third World women as a function of political and economic interests, embodied in a male-dominated, U.S.-sponsored international population control effort directed primarily at women.[2] It would be reasonable to conclude from Hartmann's study that the gap between middle-class women in the United States and Third World women who are direct targets of population control efforts is wide. When considered by itself, my own study of the professional literature also supports that view. The data derived from interviewing women of various social circumstances within the United States, however, complicates that picture. Women in the United States have received some of the same dangerous products from the same class of professionals with the same tragic results in terms of their reproductive and sexual health.

How do we account for those similarities between women when other differences are so apparent?

The feminist literature dealing with the relationship between the medical system and sexuality in the United States offers some insight into the shared circumstances of women of different classes and races. Gena Corea's work is particularly useful in that respect. Corea views class and race oppression as functions of gender oppression. The increasing control over reproductive technologies by professionals who are men threatens to force women into new forms of servitude. According to Corea, men's efforts to control women's fertility originate not from the economic interests of men or couples, but from the male's innate alienation from the processes and products of reproduction.

Corea argues that men, through their hegemony within the medical system, assert their power and authority over women in the interest of controlling women's reproductive capacities and taking over the production of children. The strength of Corea's work is in her documentation of the erosion of women's autonomy by physicians and scientists— a problem common to women of all classes and races in her examples. Corea does not, however, explain differences among men. While the majority of physicians and scientists coming into contact with women through the health care system are men, the majority of men are not physicians and scientists. The majority of men, in fact, come into contact with the medical profession in a position not entirely unlike the position of women vis-à-vis that profession. The physician-patient relationship is more often than not a potentially dangerous and degrading power relationship in which the patient, regardless of gender, is the vulnerable subordinate. And it is not at all clear that the actions of professional men vis-à-vis women are in any way supportive of the interests of men in women's personal lives—as husbands or as fathers of the children medical science seems to be trying to expropriate. To the extent that the actions of professionals represent class or racial interests in addition to gender interests, it is reasonable to suppose that the interests of professional men conflict with the interests of disadvantaged men just as they do with disadvantaged women. Differences among men pose a serious challenge to Corea's biological determinist perspective.[3]

Andrea Dworkin also offers an explanation for women's sexual oppression in terms of biological determinism. But for Dworkin, the subjugation of women occurs prior to any consideration of parenthood. It is intercourse, Dworkin believes, that explains the subjugation of women—and all other forms of social oppression. Dworkin blames God, not men, for the biologically determined inferior status of women. Dworkin wrote, "The rules of intercourse are intended to keep people away from the slippery slope God appears to dislike most: a lessening of differences between the sexes, the conflation of male and female natures into one human nature." Law and society, Dworkin believes, have been shaped to protect men, as a class. Dworkin locates the basis of political life in personal sexual relations, and she credits men, not feminists, with the insight that the personal is political: "The principle that 'the personal is political' belongs to patriarchal law itself, originating there in a virtual synthesis of intimacy and state policy, the private and the public, the penis and the rule of men."[4]

The foundation of Dworkin's theoretical point is that the very act of intercourse is an act of possession, an invasion of privacy, the literal penetration of the integrity of a woman's body. Dworkin recognizes but discounts attempts by feminists to imagine that intercourse could be fundamentally different in the context of egalitarian sexual relationships.[5] Surprisingly, she ignores one material condition supporting her analysis that something inherent in the act of intercourse is inevitably oppressive to women: Intercourse, after all, exposes women to pregnancy. It also brings about the need for contraception and abortion. As long as intercourse entails any risk of pregnancy when pregnancy is not desired, it is a source of potentially severe, even deadly, risk for women. It might be reasonable to argue that the material consequence of intercourse makes a consideration of its cultural primacy vital in the study of the ontology of sexual oppression. But Dworkin does not make that argument. In her view, anatomy is destiny, and no form of social change can intervene to alter that fact.

Barbara Ehrenreich views the agency of men as more decisive in determining the conditions of women's lives. Ehrenreich divides men into two spheres of influence, public and private. From the public sphere, men control women's lives through their expertise, dispensing advice on which women have become dependent for the conduct of their personal lives. In the private sphere, men as would-be or erstwhile partners control the conditions of women's lives by a "flight from responsibility" that has left women with crushing economic and domestic burdens. The condition of women has become more universal, Ehrenreich believes, as women have been forced to work for very low wages, to pay for the support of children, including day care, or to live on welfare.[6]

Within feminism, a conservative trend is developing among women who believe that the present conditions women face have less to do with men in personal life than with economic and political issues women share with men. Germaine Greer has argued that the answer to the attack by population control forces on Third World women is the strengthening of family as a locus of women's resistance. The restoration of matrifocal female support networks (within the patriarchal family structure), she believes, promises to give women the opportunity to escape external control over their personal lives and procreative capacities.[7]

Unlike Ehrenreich, who places the burden of necessary social change on the shoulders of men, whom she believes must act more responsibly in their personal relationships with women, Greer argues for a suspension of sexual politics in the interest of building strong families. Greer is joined in her call to strengthen the family by Betty Friedan, who thinks that feminism must "transcend female/male polarization" in order to achieve "the new human wholeness that is the promise of feminism." Calling the new "conservative pro-family feminism" a "Great Leap Backward," Judith Stacey criticizes Greer and Friedan for wanting to "maintain . . . sexual equality as a vague futuristic goal" while seeking to "curtail explicitly feminist struggle to achieve it."[8]

This argument among feminists arises from different perspectives about the nature of the separate sphere inhabited by women. Radical feminists view the sphere of women and the sphere of men as two distinct entities or experiences, whether caused by men or God, by economy, polity, or nature. More conservative feminists see the two spheres as public and private. Men inhabit both spheres, and their relationship to women is fundamentally different in each. In each paradigm the unity of women within a common sphere is assumed but not clearly demonstrated or explained.

In a recent essay Linda Kerber discussed the history of social thought regarding the metaphor of separate spheres. She pointed out that the metaphor has been used rather loosely to refer symbolically to spheres of influence or experience and literally to refer to physical locations of activity. Modern social change has challenged the concept of separate spheres. In both a symbolic and a literal sense, men and women seem to share more space. There appears to be a breakdown of the boundaries between genders, with men and women sharing the workplace, the care of the home, the ownership of property, and the care and custody of children. Kerber wrote, "The metaphor [of separate spheres] remains resonant because it retains some superficial vitality. For all that men's 'spheres' and women's 'spheres' now overlap, vast areas of our experience and consciousness do not overlap. The boundaries may be fuzzier but our private spaces and our public spaces are still in many important senses gendered."[9]

In Heidi Hartmann's view, separate spheres remain salient but do not indicate a static subjugation of women within a fundamentally oppressive sphere. According to Hartmann, women have become more autonomous in recent decades. She wrote, "On the whole, economic changes of the past several decades have been positive for women. Women in advanced industrialized countries today have more access to economic resources independently of men than ever before in human history. They have more control over the conditions of their lives, and probably have a higher standard of living relative to men than at any time previously."[10]

Hartmann identified a number of demographic changes that have influenced women's autonomy since the 1950s. Marriage has become more universal, but marriages are delayed; childbirth has also become more universal, but it, too, is being delayed; women are having fewer children, and the children are spaced closer together, so fewer years of a woman's life are being spent in active mothering; divorce is more prevalent; women head more households; and women spend more time living alone, rather than with parents or husbands. Hartmann wrote, "The experience of marriage and childbearing have become more universal for women over the course of the twentieth century (and for childbearing, particularly since 1940), but as fertility has fallen and divorce has increased, living in families and raising children has become limited to a shorter period of the average woman's life. A substantial and increasing proportion of women raise children in households that do not include a husband or male partner."[11]

Hartmann disagrees with Ehrenreich that these changes have impoverished women. She points out that poor women living alone or as heads of households were more often than not impoverished before they left or were left by men.[12]

> One response to all these changes is to certify a family crisis and to bemoan the increased exploitation of women who must support households and children on their own or who bear the brunt of speed-up that occurs when both adults must work outside the home. But another interpretation, one that I support, is to see these changes as largely positive for women because they contribute to women's increased autonomy from men and their increased economic independence, whether or not they live with men.[13]

My study of the case of the Dalkon Shield strongly suggests that the concept of separate spheres remains resonant, and that women's sphere is now related to women's autonomy at the same time that it continues to embody aspects of women's oppression. As women have gained economic independence from men in personal life, women have become more dependent on health professionals. In the area of reproductive health, women's sphere is a gendered sphere, because women's bodies bear the consequences of sexuality as we define and experience it.

To a great extent, consideration of men's roles in their personal lives was lacking in women's testimonies about their procreative decisions. When considering why they used particular methods of contraception, some women referred to men's lack of cooperation, but few saw the actions of sexual partners as decisive. Often the mention of male responsibility or the wish that an effective method would be developed for men was made in retrospect. None of the women said that they had wanted men to use condoms at the time that they chose to use the Dalkon Shield. Only after the fact did women often wish they had made another choice, or that their partners had.

The focus of women's discussions was outside the home or the bedroom. The sphere of greatest importance in these women's stories was the gynecologist's office, the family planning clinic, the hospital, the examining table, and the operating room. The relationships of women to health care professionals overshadowed their relationships to their sexual partners in their narratives so far that the sexual relationship became almost entirely separate from its procreative contingencies.

Some might argue that men's "flight from responsibility" put women in that position in the first place, but these women did not see it that way. All the women interviewed said that they felt it was their responsibility to use contraception. While some women expressed some ambivalence about the burden of that responsibility being exclusively their own, other women clearly and emphatically stated that they *wanted* that responsibility.

Times had changed. In the midnineteenth century, children had already become a liability for middle-class husbands who aspired to increase their economic and social status through accumulation of property. Children ceased to be economic assets once they no longer helped to produce income through family farming and domestic labor. For middle-class women, however, children had not become unambiguously burdensome. Middle-class women usually did not leave the home to work, and within the home they often had servants to help them care for children. At that time it may well have been men, not women, who most aggressively sought to decrease family size.

By the 1960s, however, women could not rely on a husband's wage for support. Economic security for middle-class women depended on women's own wages in several ways. Many women were staying single longer or were living alone or as heads of households, as Heidi Hartmann pointed out. Most women no longer had hired domestic help to care for dependent children. Most children were no longer economic assets at any time in their parents' lives. Economic security was no longer available to aging parents through their children; it was provided, however inadequately, through the state. The size of the Social Security check would depend on the wages earned over the lifespan. Supplementary retirement programs depended on continuity of work, as well as the size of the paycheck. Day care was often unavailable, and most centers would not accept children under the age of two. Most women would have to take at least two years off from work for every child born. Day care was often prohibitively expensive as well, severely reducing the earnings of working parents. To have children meant to interrupt careers or severely diminish economic resources, or both.

As Heidi Hartmann suggested, economic autonomy can be a precondition for a more general independence in women's lives. Unplanned or untimely pregnancies can threaten women's economic independence. Women who must stay home to care for babies become dependent on the wages of individual men or on the welfare state. Women who continue to work and who must pay for day care can lose their entire paychecks to those costs. Just as economic autonomy can be a precondition for independence in other areas of life, economic dependence can be the precondition for the overall curtailment of women's freedom. Women lose status in the job market, they lose buying power as consumers, and it might be reasonable to suggest that many women lose leverage within personal relationships when economic security is provided for the entire family by the man's wages alone.

While the sample of women interviewed for this project is not meant to be representative of the larger population of women for whom these issues are relevant, it might be useful to note here that only one of those women was unemployed, and she was the woman who reported having the least control over her life within her family and her marriage. She said that her husband would not "allow" her to work. He opposed her desire to continue her education, even to complete high school equivalency requirements. She was an artistically talented woman who wanted a career of her own. She said that she had never used birth control (although she had in fact tried a variety of methods), and she had four children and some serious pregnancy-related health problems. She was concerned with the number of children she had only because of her own and her children's health problems and because her husband had to work so hard. She wanted her husband to have a vasectomy, but he refused. She then had a tubal ligation which she said had been performed with her permission but against her will. She was the only still-married woman in the sample who reported that she was physically battered by her husband.

All the other women were either employed full time or were students. The two women who were students were employed part time. All emphatically stated that they chose methods of birth control that they believed would absolutely protect them from pregnancy. They were willing to endure agonizing pain to secure their autonomy by controlling their procreative power. They often suspended concern for their physical safety in order to assure that they would be safe from the consequences of pregnancy. Each woman, in her own way, said that an unplanned pregnancy would have meant disaster. Many of the women spoke eloquently about the degree to which unplanned pregnancies had already altered their lives.

Demographers have found that women who have some autonomy in their lives prefer to have fewer children. The more education she has, the fewer children a woman will want; if she works after marriage, the same correlation applies. According to Berent, "The data . . . confirm that working women have fewer children than non-working women, and that the strength of this association varies positively with the length of employment since marriage in relation to marriage duration."[14] It seems reasonable to view this as a dialectical relationship. Women who work and women who attain higher levels of education have fewer children; and women who have fewer children can continue to work and can attain higher levels of education.

It might be reasonable to argue that women did not have to turn to the medical profession to obtain contraceptive products or to use methods that were effective. Condoms could have been used alone or in combination with spermicides or calendar rhythm to obtain effectiveness equal to or greater than that promised by oral contraceptives and IUDs. But the pill and the IUD offered women something women said they thought they wanted—the final step in making reproduction and sexuality two entirely separate considerations. With the necessities of birth control separated from the time and place of coitus, a new kind of freedom—"spontaneity"—was possible. As one woman said, the old-fashioned condom was a joke at the time that she used the Dalkon Shield. That sentiment was shared by several of the women. At the same time, professionals whose economic interests were vested in modern products promoted the idea that old-fashioned methods were undesirable not only because they interfered with spontaneity and tended to be inconvenient or messy to use, but also because they were allegedly less effective than more modern products.

Women who used the Dalkon Shield generally believed that they were acting on their own behalf, protecting themselves by choosing a scientifically developed and carefully tested product or by relying on physicians to choose such a product for them. The results were unexpected. Women who described themselves as emancipated, who made educated and informed decisions, who were proud of their ability to plan their lives and steer their own destinies effectively, thought that they had escaped the traditional separate sphere of women's oppression. Many were working in a world previously reserved for men, and they were making it in that world on their own—without the help of parents, and often without the help of spouses. Their experiences with the Dalkon Shield—and with other contraceptives that injured them—drew them back into the traditional female aspects of experience, where they formed or renewed bonds with women whose lives they had once rejected. Fully realized autonomy was not possible for these women because the social context within which they sought to achieve that autonomy was fundamentally oppressive.

Women's experiences may be becoming more universal in two respects. First, women may be becoming more autonomous in personal life, and that autonomy in some ways makes the experiences of men and women who share aspects of their social lives with each other more similar. In terms of procreative issues, as the literal sphere of reproductive control continues to pass to professionals in the laboratory, the corporation, the state, the physician's office, and the hospital, the bodies of men may become targets in efforts that have more to do with class, race, and politics than with gender. Second, as the control of women's procreative capacities passes increasingly to the same authorities, the experiences of women across the boundaries of class, race, and country may become more universal.

The outcome of these changes cannot be predicted. Increased autonomy for women may give some leverage for restructuring personal life and sexual politics. A woman with an income and a life of her own can perhaps say no to relationships that jeopardize her autonomy, her health, and her vitality. For the first time in recorded history, women's bodies are beginning to belong to women. The feminist demand for the right to bodily integrity to be recognized in law has coincided with the historical transformation of women's economic sphere.

As women increasingly share experiences that transcend the boundaries of class and race, the potential for unity in action among women may also increase. Real alternatives to the old patriarchal forms of dependency could result from women's organizing to bring about mutually beneficial change. As women of all classes command more economic resources, the need individually or collectively to "go back home" to the patriarchal family may diminish.

It remains to be seen whether these trends toward shared concerns will lead to unity in action to bring about social change that will benefit the majority of people, or whether new forms of privilege and oppression will emerge to replace the old. A great deal may depend on the emerging meaning of autonomy and its relationship to social responsibility. If autonomy for women means nothing more than the opportunity to develop individualism, it will hold little promise for the majority of people. Modern surrogate motherhood stands as a meaningful example of the ways in which the freedom of one woman can be bought at the expense of another. One woman can now buy what another woman has to sell—the use of her body for the purpose of reproduction. While some women own their own bodies for the first time, other women have little else to sell but their "labor" power—literally.

As men share more of the material conditions of life with women of their own classes and races, it is possible that shared interests will lead to unity in action to bring about mutually beneficial social change. Many men, having already historically lost control over women in their personal lives, may now have more to gain from concession and cooperation than from oppression of women. It is possible that personal relationships (and families) could become important havens of resistance against the power of the corporation, the medical profession, and the potentially repressive state if those relationships are transformed by sexual politics into egalitarian and democratic forms.

For the transformations that we are witnessing to lead to freedom for women from sexual oppression, it is necessary that social change be guided by an explicitly feminist agenda, with sexual politics at its core and social responsibility as its essence. A feminist transformation of sexuality could have radical implications for women and for all oppressed people. The feminist demand for socially responsible sexuality—for "safe sex" for women—is at heart a demand for an ethical social world. It is not a libertarian demand for individualism, but a demand for social justice. As ethicist Beverly Wildung Harrison wrote, "No concern for social justice is genuine if it does not lie close to concrete historical consequences."[15] This study has been about the concrete historical consequences for potentially fertile women of heterosexuality practiced in a particular way. Because coitus is essential to "normal" heterosexuality in our culture, birth control is necessary for sex to be possible without procreative consequences. The availability of birth control is thus viewed as liberating because it allows the free enjoyment of sex.

For women who have been injured by birth control methods, the promised liberation to enjoy sex has proved elusive. For many women, sex itself has been altered or destroyed by injuries. A great deal of attention is given to the destruction of reproductive functions by scarring or by surgical removal of the uterus after injury. But loss of sexual functions is also a consequence. Women who have pelvic adhesions as the result of infection have a chronic problem with pain and with the potential for tearing of affected tissue. Orgasm, as one young woman in this study pointed out, can become too painful to endure if pelvic contractions cause adhesions to pull and tear. The loss of the uterus is another injury to sexual function. The uterus is a vital organ in orgasmic response. The fact that the clitoris is the primary organ in sexual stimulation obscures the fact that the entire pelvic region is involved. Engorgement and contractions of the uterus during orgasm intensify the pleasure. When the uterus is removed orgasm remains possible, but the feelings are altered by the absence of the deep pelvic sensations that normally are felt in that part of the body. Any method of birth control that makes women too sick to enjoy sex is a dubious means to sexual liberation.

Risks associated with heterosexuality for women fall into three categories. The first is the risk of disease; the second is the risk of pregnancy; and the third is the risk of injury as a consequence of efforts to curtail procreative power. Women often exchange one risk for another. We can trade the risk of pregnancy for the risk of contraceptive injury, or vice versa. When we must choose among available contraceptive methods we trade effectiveness against safety. Abstinence is viewed as the only alternative to this trading of one risk for another. However, although abstinence is certainly safe, it is not safe *sex*.

Anthropologist Mina Davis Caulfield has suggested that the most natural aspect of human sexuality is our ability, as a species, to create our own sexual nature. Human sexuality is a product of human cultures. We literally *make* love. Unlike other primates, humans are not constrained by estrus cycles that regulate sexual response or instincts that govern sexual style. Our sexuality, Caulfield wrote, "is much more than a means of producing offspring; in every known society, it is invested with deep symbolic meaning."[16] A consideration of the symbolic meaning and social construction of sexual norms in our own culture may help us to evaluate the extent of our power to diminish or eliminate risks.

Sex is never safe for women who must trade one set of risks for an-other. But sex can be made safer for women if attention is given to the range of human potential in shaping the way we make love. The least risky means of sexual expression are those that avoid penetration and/or the exchange of body fluids. This is so whether the risks are associated with pregnancy or disease. Couples who wish to enjoy orgasmic sex and want to minimize the risks of disease, pregnancy, or birth control inju-ries have the option of mutual manual stimulation. This means absti-nence from coitus, but not abstinence from sex. Couples who prefer coitus have the option to use natural birth control to time fertility, and can minimize the chance of pregnancy by limiting coitus to times when they are reasonably sure that the woman is not fertile and then using barrier methods just in case they have miscalculated. Using two barrier methods at the same time, for instance a diaphragm and a condom, gives protection equal to that associated with hormonal contraceptives and IUDs. The major drawback for couples using this second set of options is that sexual pleasure may be diminished with the use of barrier methods, a problem not associated with manual sex. Oral sex and pen-etration of parts of the body other than the vagina are options that avoid the risk of pregnancy but retain the risk of disease, including AIDS.

So little attention has been given to the study of sexuality in the social sciences that we have little knowledge or insight into how or why coitus has persisted as the defining norm of heterosexual expression despite its many consequences. Perhaps long ago human survival depended on procreation to the extent that societies defined other forms of expression as deviant. But in modern times, procreation without limit has been a problem of such magnitude that billions risk their lives and health to attempt to circumvent it. If coitus were the most pleasurable means of sexual expression for men or women, that might provide the answer to the question of its persistence; but even this has been drawn into ques-tion by feminists, sex researchers, and men's popular culture in the twentieth century. The anatomy of women's sexuality makes the least risky sexual style, manual stimulation, more conducive to orgasm than coitus. Many men have reported to sex researchers that manual sex is the most pleasurable for them as well. It is of historical importance that "going all the way" in our culture has not meant the experience of orgasm, but the experience of coitus even in the absence of orgasm. Many women have risked their lives for a form of sexual expression that has given them no pleasure. Both men and women have shouldered economic and social burdens associated with untimely pregnancy as a consequence of the assumption that normal heterosexual sex must involve coitus.

At the present time, when safe sex is such an important issue for all of us and when so many risks derive from the actions of the state, the corporations, and the medical profession, it is imperative that we critically examine the social construction of sexual norms and include all our options in our risk/benefit analysis of alternative sexual choices. With the experiences of men and women becoming more universal in terms of the details of personal life, the potential of individual couples to resist collective risks could be enhanced. Actions of the state that might otherwise limit our choices, and irresponsible actions by corporate or medical personnel, could be rendered less harmful to us if we become willing to reshape sexual norms in our own interest. We have the choice and the power to shape sexuality to be more conducive to our safety and our free enjoyment of our human sexual potential, unhampered by nature, by the limitations of technology and scientific knowledge, or by the intrusive interests of experts, policy makers and profiteers. Individual answers alone cannot substitute for collective solutions. But individual resistance that protects our health, our lives, and our autonomy can set the stage for collective resistance and progressive social change.

Epilogue

In 1991 a paper in the *Journal of Clinical Epidemiology* claimed that the link that had previously been established between intrauterine devices and pelvic inflammatory disease was based on a methodologically flawed study. The paper, "The Intrauterine Device and Pelvic Inflammatory Disease: The Women's Health Study Reanalyzed," was not a new study of IUDs; it merely purported to reanalyze data published in the 1981 Women's Health Study. The Women's Health Study had claimed that women using IUDs were more likely than a control group to suffer a first incidence of pelvic inflammatory disease.

The findings of the 1991 paper were, however, reported in the national news as though they were the result of a new study of intrauterine devices, not simply a methodological critique of an older study. The potential consumer was once again offered false assurances that some women, at least, could safely use intrauterine devices. The paper—and the media reports that followed it—also claimed that these new findings indicated that the Dalkon Shield had not been the cause of the infections linked to it. The demise of the A. H. Robins Corporation, the authors maintained, had resulted from the acceptance by the courts of results from a single flawed study.

Two of the three authors of the paper had once acted as expert witnesses in defense of A. H. Robins in the Dalkon Shield case. To their credit, they disclosed that fact in a note to readers published at the beginning of their paper. The authors stated that they had completed their reanalysis in October 1983 and had offered their findings to A. H. Robins. The company, they asserted, never used their reanalysis in the courtroom because they "had already decided that continued defense of the Dalkon Shield was hopeless."

That claim alone strains the credibility of the paper and its authors. The continued efforts of A. H. Robins to avoid accountability in the Dalkon Shield case and to discredit litigants long after October 1983 is a matter of public record. If the reanalysis of the Women's Health Study data could have withstood the scrutiny it would have been subject to in court, during litigation, it is reasonable to assume that the company's attorneys would have used it. The authors' statement that they withheld their findings until after the case was settled in order to avoid charges that they were publishing the paper for economic gain is also suspect, particularly given recent trends to reintroduce IUDs in the United States.

There are more serious problems with the paper, however. First, the authors address only one case-control study; many other studies, using various methods, have linked IUDs with infection. Second, they address only infection as a danger of IUD use; the Women's Health Study and many other studies have linked the IUD to many serious side effects in addition to pelvic inflammatory disease. Third, they limited their discussion to sexually transmitted infectious organisms. Fourth, in character with A. H. Robins' consistent efforts to blame the victims for their injuries, the authors speculate that IUD users, as a group, may be more promiscuous, less religious, less informed (but more influenced by the media), more likely to engage in risky behavior, more likely to be socioeconomically disadvantaged, and less likely to consult physicians in a timely manner when they have an infection (but more likely to make complaints to physicians that lead to false-positive diagnoses when they don't have infections) than women who do not use IUDs. Any increase in infections that might appear among these women, according to the authors' speculation, could be attributed to their unique demographic characteristics and their own behavior rather than to the intrauterine device. Fifth, the authors neither test their hypotheses themselves nor cite studies to support their speculations.

The 1981 Women's Health Study compared IUD users with women who used other methods of contraception, including barrier methods and the pill. The authors who reanalyzed that study claimed that because the pill and barrier methods are thought to protect against pelvic inflammatory disease, users of IUDs should have been compared to noncontraceptors. They claimed that any significant difference between incidence of pelvic inflammatory disease in IUD users and in contraceptors using other methods was due not to an increase in PID in IUD users, but to a decrease in PID among users of the other methods. For the prospective consumer, this is curious logic. What woman is likely to consider not contracepting as an alternative to IUD use? If barrier methods or oral contraceptives may decrease the chances of developing PID when compared to intrauterine devices, most women considering using an IUD will want to know this.

Most seriously, the authors failed to evaluate or acknowledge studies showing that IUD-related infections may be introduced to the uterus through the woman's own bloodstream, studies showing that the IUD creates an ecological niche perfect for the harboring and growth of bacteria, and studies identifying blood-borne bacteria as typical in IUD-related pelvic inflammatory disease.

If the authors' critique of the Women's Health Study had conclusively shown that study to be completely invalid, which it did not, it still would not indicate that IUDs are safe, or that they do not cause infections. It would merely indicate that the original study could not offer any answers to questions about the link between IUDs and pelvic infections.

The publicity given the reanalysis of the Women's Health Study is reminiscent of the misinformation that pervaded the media throughout the Dalkon Shield case. The consumer is likely to be treated to more confusion in the months and years to come as (1) the FDA plans another study of intrauterine devices, (2) the debate over the safety of the newly approved implantable contraceptive Norplant continues, and (3) new contraceptive products—for men and women—are introduced. The words of one of the women I interviewed offer an important reminder as we struggle in a sea of misinformation to inform ourselves and make responsible decisions about our health, our procreative power, and our sexuality: "It's not a matter of being an informed consumer; it's a matter of being a cynic to save your life."

Notes

Introduction

1. Barney Glaser and Anselm Strauss, *The Discovery of Grounded Theory*. Chicago: Aldine, 1967.

Chapter 1

1. Paul Starr, *The Transformation of American Medicine* (New York: Basic Books, 1982), esp. 52, 82, 88.

2. Ibid., 69–70, 40.

3. Ibid., 20, 142.

4. Ibid., 129.

5. Barbara Ehrenreich and Dierdre English, *Witches, Midwives and Nurses: A History of Women Healers* (Old Westbury, N.Y.: Feminist Press, 1973).

6. Kristin Luker, *Abortion and the Politics of Motherhood* (Berkeley: University of California Press, 1984), 266 n. 13. The issue of men's willingness to cooperate with women rather than merely to dominate them in matters related to contraception is debated. Luker claims that in the nineteenth century, it appeared that men knew about and supported women's decisions to obtain abortions, although the initiative for obtaining one was left to the woman in most cases.

7. Ibid., 68.

8. James C. Mohr, *Abortion in America: The Origins and Evolution of National Policy, 1800–1900* (New York: Oxford University Press, 1978), 86, 91, 110–11, 115.

9. Ibid., 113.

10. Linda Gordon, *Woman's Body, Woman's Right* (New York: Penguin, 1977).

11. Stephen J. Gould, *The Mismeasure of Man* (New York: W.W. Norton, 1981).

12. Gordon, *Woman's Body*, 21, 49, 319.

13. Ibid., 351–52.

14. Heidi Hartmann, "Changes in Women's Economic and Family Roles in Post–World War II United States," in *Women, Households and the Economy*, ed. Lourdes Beneira and Catherine A. Stimpson (New Brunswick: Rutgers University Press, 1987), 33–64.

15. Jerzy Berent, "Family Size Preference in Europe and U.S.A.: Ultimate Expected Number of Children," *World Fertility Surveys* (1983): 27.

16. H. Hartmann, "Changes in Women's Economic and Family Roles," 45.

17. Barbara Seaman, *The Doctors' Case against the Pill*, rev. ed. (Garden City, N.Y.: Doubleday, 1980), 75.

18. John Rock, "The Significance of Population Research," in *Population Research* (Washington: PCC, 1971).

19. Boston Women's Health Collective, *The New Our Bodies, Ourselves* (New York: Simon and Schuster, 1984), 228.

20. Norman Himes, *Medical History of Contraception* (New York: Gamut, 1963), introduction, 4.

21. Ibid., 17–18, 25.

22. Ibid., 109, 177.

23. Lucile F. Newman, ed., *Women's Medicine: A Cross-Cultural Study of Indigenous Fertility Regulation* (New Brunswick: Rutgers University Press, 1985), 181.

24. See Browner's discussion of Cali, Colombia, and Sukkary-Stolba's discussion of two Egyptian villages, both in *Women's Medicine*, ed. Lucile F. Newman, 78–97, 99–123.

25. Newman, *Women's Medicine*, 183–84.

26. This problem occurs in many cultures. It usually involves methods of abortion, including violence to the external body—usually the abdomen or back—or the oral or intravaginal intake of toxic substances.

27. See Newman, *Women's Medicine*, for discussions of these issues that are culture specific.

28. Gordon, *Woman's Body*, 403.

29. Boston Women's Health Collective, *The New Our Bodies, Ourselves*, 309.

30. Ibid., 310.

31. Diane Scully, *Men Who Control Women's Health: The Miseducation of Obstetrician-Gynecologists* (Boston: Houghton Mifflin, 1980), 43–44.

32. Barbara Seaman, "Tell Me Doctor: 'Why Did Birth Control Fail Me?'" *Ladies' Home Journal*, November 1965, 167.

33. Laurence Lader, "Why Birth Control Fails." *McCall's*, October 1969, 163.

34. Garrett Hardin, *Birth Control* (New York: Pegasus, 1970), 135.

35. U.S. Food and Drug Administration, Advisory Committee on Obstetrics and Gynecology, *Report on Oral Contraceptives* (1966 [Document No. 228-677-66-2]), 1.

36. Ibid., 2.

37. Ibid., 6.

38. Ibid., 6–8.

39. Ibid., 9–10.

40. Ibid., 10.

41. Ibid., 11–12.

42. Ibid., 12–13.

43. Ibid., 1.

44. U.S. Food and Drug Administration, Advisory Committee on Obstetrics and Gynecology, *Second Report on Oral Contraceptives* (August 1, 1969 [Document No. 362-666-0-69-2]), 13.

45. Idem, *Report on Intrauterine Devices* (1968 [Document No. 290-137 0-68-3]), 1.

46. Joyce Avrech Berkman, "Historical Styles of Contraceptive Advocacy," in *Birth Control and Controlling Birth: Woman-Centered Perspectives*, ed. Helen B. Holmes, Betty B. Hoskins, and Michael Gross (Clifton, N.J.: Humana, 1980), 31.

47. Beverly Wildung Harrison, *Our Right to Choose: Toward a New Ethic of Abortion* (Boston: Beacon, 1983).

48. U.S. FDA, *Report on Intrauterine Devices*, 17.

49. Ibid., 25, 28.

50. Ibid., 30, 31, 32.

51. Ibid., 35–37.

52. Ibid., 40.

53. Carol Korenbrat, "Value Conflicts in Biomedical Research into Future Contraceptives," in *Birth Control and Controlling Birth*, ed. Holmes, Hoskins, and Gross, 47–48.

54. U.S. FDA, *Second Report on Oral Contraceptives*, 1.

55. Ibid., 2.

56. Ibid., 8.

57. Ibid., 8–9.

58. U.S. Congress, Senate, Select Committee on Small Business, Subcommittee on Monopoly, *Present Status of Competition in the Pharmaceutical Industry* (91st Cong., 2d sess., 1970, [Document No. 40-471-70]), 5921–22.

59. Ibid., 5922.

60. Ibid., 5924–25.

61. Ibid., 5925.

62. Ibid., 5227–28.

63. Ibid., 5926.

64. Ibid., 7314.

65. Ibid., 6137.

66. Ibid., 6140.

67. Ibid., 6142.

68. Ibid., 6053.

69. Ibid., 6058.

70. Ibid., 6817–18.

71. Ibid.

72. *Time,* May 2, 1970, 58.

73. Morton Mintz, *The Pill: An Alarming Report* (Boston: Beacon, 1969), 118.

74. Paul Vaughan, *The Pill on Trial* (New York: Coward-McCann, 1970), 63, 66.

75. Alan F. Guttmacher, *Birth Control and Love: The Complete Guide to Contraception and Fertility* (London: Macmillan, 1969).

76. Ibid., 33, 34.

77. Ibid., 7, 137.

Chapter 2

1. Sybil Shainwald, "The Story of the Dalkon Shield," in *The Dalkon Shield,* ed. Sybil Shainwald (Washington: NWHN, 1985), 8.

2. Ibid.

3. Morton Mintz, *At Any Cost: Corporate Greed, Women, and the Dalkon Shield* (New York: Pantheon, 1985), 28.

4. Roger B. Scott, "Critical Illnesses and Deaths Associated with Intrauterine Devices," *Obstetrics and Gynecology* 31 (1968): 322–26.

5. U.S. Food and Drug Administration, Advisory Committee on Obstetrics and Gynecology, *Report on Intrauterine Devices* (1968 [Document No. 290-137 0-68-2]), 8–9.

6. J. Robert Willson and William J. Ledger, "Complications Associated with the

Use of Intrauterine Contraceptive Devices in Women of Middle and Upper Socio-economic Class," *American Journal of Obstetrics and Gynecology* 100 (1968): 649.

7. William J. Ledger and Frank G. Schrader, "Death from Septicemia Following Insertion of an Intrauterine Contraceptive Device: Report of a Case," *Obstetrics and Gynecology* 31 (1968): 846–47.

8. Charles H. Birnberg and Michael S. Burnhill, "Whither the IUD? The Present and Future of Intrauterine Contraceptives," *Obstetrics and Gynecology* 31 (1968): 862.

9. George J. Solish and Gregory Majzlin, "New Stainless Steel Spring for Intrauterine Contraception," *Obstetrics and Gynecology* 32 (1968): 116–19, 862.

10. Mogens Osler and Paul E. Lebech, "A New Form of Intrauterine Device," *American Journal of Obstetrics and Gynecology* 102 (1968): 1175–76; Hugh J. Davis, *Intrauterine Devices for Contraception: The IUD* (Baltimore: Williams and Wilkins, 1971), 153–66.

11. C. Irving Meeker, "Use of Drugs and Intrauterine Devices for Birth Control," *New England Journal of Medicine* 28 (1969): 1058–60.

12. Kamla Dhall, G. I. Dhall, and Brij Bala Gupta, "Uterine Perforation with the Lippes Loop: Detection by Hysterography," *Obstetrics and Gynecology* 34 (1969): 266–70.

13. H. Robert Misenhimer and Rafael Garcia-Bunuel, "Failure of Intrauterine Contraceptive Devices and Fungal Infection in the Fetus," *Obstetrics and Gynecology* 34 (1969): 368–72.

14. Jaime A. Zipper et al., "Metallic Copper as an Intrauterine Contraceptive Adjunct to the 'T' Device," *American Journal of Obstetrics and Gynecology* 105 (1969): 1274; Hugh J. Davis, *Intrauterine Devices*, 164, 165.

15. U.S. Congress, Senate, Select Committee on Small Business, Subcommittee on Monopoly, *Present Status of Competition in the Pharmaceutical Industry* (91st Cong., 2d sess., 1970 [Document No. 40-471-70]), 5926–28.

16. Ibid., 5926, 5935, 5936.

17. Ibid., 5939, 5941. This reference by Davis to meningitis turned out to be ironic; litigation was brought against the manufacturer of the Dalkon Shield several years later on behalf of a young girl who developed fetal meningitis while in utero with a Dalkon Shield. See the *Wall Street Journal* (March 17, 1980), 19, "A. H. Robins Co. Pays $1.4 Million to Settle Contraceptive Suit."

18. U.S. Congress, *Competition in the Pharmaceutical Industry*, 5941.

19. Hugh J. Davis, "The Shield Intrauterine Device: A Superior Modern Contraceptive," *American Journal of Obstetrics and Gynecology* 106 (1970): 455–56.

20. "Virtually Failsafe IUD Seen in Year," *Journal of the American Medical Association* 212 (1970): 1136; Mintz, *At Any Cost*, 64.

21. Shainwald, "The Story of the Dalkon Shield," 10–12. Also see Mintz, *At Any Cost*, 58–59; and Susan Perry and Jim Dawson, *Nightmare: Women and the Dalkon Shield* (New York: Macmillan, 1985), 243–44.

22. Hugh J. Davis and John Lesinski, "Mechanisms of Action of Intrauterine Contraceptives in Women," *Obstetrics and Gynecology* 36 (1970): 352, 357.

23. Mintz, *At Any Cost*, 103–4; Shainwald, "The Story of the Dalkon Shield," 11–12, 13.

24. R. P. Bernard, "Factors Governing IUD Performance," *American Journal of Public Health* 61 (1971): 559; Shainwald, "The Story of the Dalkon Shield," 13.

25. Mintz, *At Any Cost*, 99.

26. Davis, *Intrauterine Devices*, v.

27. Ibid., 33, 34–35, 46–47.

28. Mintz, *At Any Cost*, 126–27.

29. Davis, *Intrauterine Devices*, 60–61, 79.

30. Ibid., 82.

31. Ibid., 92, 94.

32. Ibid., 106.

33. Ibid., 107, 116.

34. Ibid., 151; Perry and Dawson, *Nightmare*, 73; Mintz, *At Any Cost*, 75.

35. Shainwald, "The Story of the Dalkon Shield," 12.

36. Howard J. Tatum, "Intrauterine Contraception," *American Journal of Obstetrics and Gynecology* 112 (1972): 1001.

37. Ibid., 1018–20.

38. Perry and Dawson, *Nightmare*, 104–5; "A Simple Way to Remove IUDs after Perforation," *Journal of the American Medical Association* 220 (1972): 781–82; Perry and Dawson, *Nightmare*, 97.

39. Shainwald, "The Story of the Dalkon Shield," 15.

40. Hugh J. Davis, "Intrauterine Contraceptive Devices: Present Status and Future Prospects," *American Journal of Obstetrics and Gynecology* 114 (1972): 135, 142, 149.

41. Ibid., 140, 149; Sybil Shainwald, National Women's Health Network, personal communication with author, June 21, 1986.

42. Mintz, *At Any Cost*, 9.

43. Barbara Ehrenreich, Mark Dowie, and Stephen Minkin, "The Charge: Gynocide; The Accused: The U.S. Government," *Mother Jones*, November 1979.

44. Arnold D. Sprague and Van R. Jenkins II, "Perforation of the Uterus with a Shield Intrauterine Device," *Obstetrics and Gynecology* 41 (1973): 80–81.

45. Bernard Draper and Eugene F. White, "Puerperal Insertion of the Dalkon Shield: A Private Patient Experience," *American Journal of Obstetrics and Gynecology* 115 (1973): 278–79.

46. Byrne R. Marshall, James K. Hepler, and Masaharu S. Jinguji, "Fatal Streptococcus Pyogenes Septicemia Associated with an Intrauterine Device," *Obstetrics and Gynecology* 41 (1973): 84, 86.

47. Perry and Dawson, *Nightmare*, 126, 128.

48. R. W. Jones, A. Parker, and Max Elstein, "Clinical Experience with the Dalkon Shield Intrauterine Device," *British Medical Journal*, July 1973, 145.

49. Mintz, *At Any Cost*, 189.

50. Donald R. Ostergard, "Intrauterine Contraception in Nulliparas with the Dalkon Shield," *American Journal of Obstetrics and Gynecology* 116 (1973): 108.

51. John M. Esposito, Donald M. Zaron, and George S. Zaron, "A Dalkon Shield Imbedded in a Myoma: Case Report of an Unusual Displacement of an Intrauterine Contraceptive Device," *American Journal of Obstetrics and Gynecology* 117 (1973): 580.

52. W. H. Harris, "Complications of the IUD," *Canadian Medical Journal* 119 (1973): 677.

53. "Are IUD Contraceptives Safe?" *Good Housekeeping*, October 1973, 197.

54. "Right Now: Scorecard on Birth Control," *McCall's*, November 1973, 47.

55. Boston Women's Health Collective, *Our Bodies, Ourselves: A Book by and for Women* (New York: Simon and Schuster, 1973), 121.

56. "Birth Control: A Summary and Chart of Current Contraceptive Methods," *Good Housekeeping,* February 1974, 177.

57. Johanna F. Perlmutter, "Experience with the Dalkon Shield as a Contraceptive Device," *Obstetrics and Gynecology* 43 (1974): 443, 445.

58. Kent L. Merrill, Laurence I. Burd, and Daniel J. VerBurg, "Laparoscopic Removal of Intraperitoneal Dalkon Shields: A Report of Three Cases," *American Journal of Obstetrics and Gynecology* 118 (1974): 1146–48.

59. John Newton, Julian Elias, and Anthony Johnson, "Immediate Post-Termination Insertion of Copper 7 and Dalkon Shield Intrauterine Contraceptive Devices," *Journal of Obstetrics and Gynecology of the British Commonwealth* 81 (1974): 392.

60. Robert M. Shine and Joseph F. Thompson, "The in Situ IUD and Pregnancy Outcome," *American Journal of Obstetrics and Gynecology* 119 (1974): 126, 127.

61. James Scott, response to Shine and Thompson, "In Situ IUD," *American Journal of Obstetrics and Gynecology* 119 (1974): 128–29; Vivian Gibbs, response to Shine and Thompson, "In Situ IUD," *American Journal of Obstetrics and Gynecology* 119 (1974): 129; Edward Eichner, response to Shine and Thompson, "In Situ IUD," *American Journal of Obstetrics and Gynecology* 119 (1974): 129.

62. "Robins Warns That Its IUD May Cause Severe Complications, Including Death," *Wall Street Journal,* May 29, 1974, 8; "A. H. Robins Co. Plans to Continue Marketing Its Dalkon Shield IUD," *Wall Street Journal,* May 30, 1974, 36.

63. C. D. Christian, "Maternal Deaths Associated with an Intrauterine Device," *American Journal of Obstetrics and Gynecology* 119 (1974): 441–42.

64. Ibid., 443, 444.

65. W. G. Breed, "The Efficiency of the Dalkon Shield," *Medical Journal of Australia,* June 8, 1974, 943.

66. M. D. Reefman, medical consultant at A. H. Robins in Canterbury, response to W. G. Breed, "The Efficiency of the Dalkon Shield," *Medical Journal of Australia,* June 8, 1974, 943.

67. J. S. Templeton, "Septic Abortion and the Dalkon Shield," *British Medical Journal,* June 15, 1974, 612.

68. "A. H. Robins Will Stop Sale of Dalkon Shield, Pending Safety Study," *Wall Street Journal,* June 28, 1974, 11; "Ban on Robins' IUD Becomes More Likely after New U.S. Study," *Wall Street Journal,* July 5, 1974, 15.

69. "FDA Unit Urges Ban on A. H. Robins IUD Continue until Study," *Wall Street Journal,* August 26, 1974, 14.

70. "Robins' Dalkon Shield Found No More Risky Than Other IUDs," *Wall Street Journal,* October 14, 1974, 2; "A. H. Robins Wins Clearance from FDA to Resume IUD Sale," *Wall Street Journal,* December 23, 1974, 7.

71. Russell J. Thomsen, "Pregnancy in the Presence of an Intrauterine Contraceptive Device and Amniotic Fluid Embolism: A Possible Association," *American Journal of Obstetrics and Gynecology* 121 (1975): 280.

72. Leroy R. Weekes, "Complications of Intrauterine Contraceptive Devices," *Journal of the National Medical Association* 67 (1975): 2.

73. Ibid., 2, 5, 7, 8.

74. "Are IUDs *Really* Safe?" *Good Housekeeping,* January 1975, 127.

75. "A. H. Robins to Collect Unused IUDs in U. S., Slates Modification," *Wall Street Journal,* January 21, 1975, 12.

76. Howard J. Tatum et al., "The Dalkon Shield Controversy: Structural and Bacteriological Studies of IUD Tails," *Journal of the American Medical Association* 231 (1975): 711–17.

77. Russell J. Thomsen, "Inflammatory Reaction to the Dalkon Shield," *Obstetrics and Gynecology* 46 (1975): 116.

78. "The Dalkon Shield Contraceptive Device in General Practice," *Medical Journal of Australia,* October 4, 1975, 565, 566.

79. E. Stewart Taylor et al., "The Intrauterine Device and Tubo-ovarian Abscess," *American Journal of Obstetrics and Gynecology* 123 (1975): 338, 339.

80. Philip B. Mead, Jackson B. Beecham, and John Van S. Maeck, "Incidence of Infections Associated with the Intrauterine Contraceptive Device in an Isolated Community," *American Journal of Obstetrics and Gynecology* 125 (1976): 80, 82.

81. Henry S. Kahn and Carl W. Tyler, Jr., "An Association between the Dalkon Shield and Complicated Pregnancies among Women Hospitalized for Intrauterine Contraceptive Device–Related Disorders," *American Journal of Obstetrics and Gynecology* 125 (1976): 83–86.

82. Robert Guidoin et al., "Intra-Uterine Devices: A SEM Study on the Dalkon Shield," *Biomaterials, Medical Devices and Artificial Organs: An International Journal* 4 (1976): 83–87, 114.

83. "Dalkon Shield Suits against Robins Rise, SEC Report Shows," *Wall Street Journal,* August 19, 1976, 28.

84. Terry A. Athari and Cesar Pizarro, "Perforation of the Large Bowel by a Dalkon Shield Intrauterine Device," *Journal of Reproductive Medicine* 17 (1976): 332.

85. "Statement of the National Women's Health Network on the Dalkon" (January 23, 1975), in *The Dalkon Shield,* ed. Sybil Shainwald (Washington: NWHN, 1985), 37; Ehrenreich, Dowie, and Minkin, "Gynocide."

86. Perry and Dawson, *Nightmare,* 240.

87. "Summary of Citizen's Petition: 4/25/83," in *The Dalkon Shield,* ed. Sybil Shainwald (Washington: NWHN, 1985), 438; "HHS News" (U.S. Department of Health and Human Services), in *The Dalkon Shield,* 28; "Current Trends: Pelvic Inflammatory Disease among Women Using the Dalkon Shield," *Morbidity and Mortality Weekly Report,* in *Journal of the American Medical Association* 249 (1983): 2757.

88. Harvey Bank, Marsha MacDonald, and Susan Wiechert, "Fluid Migration through the Tail of the Dalkon Shield Intrauterine Device," *Contraception* 29 (1984): 65–75.

89. Daniel K. Roberts, Douglas V. Horbelt, and Nola J. Walker, "Scanning Electron Microscopy of the Multifilament IUD String," *Contraception* 29 (1984): 215, 226–27.

90. "PPFA Clinics Advised: Remove Dalkon Shields, Prescribe Low-Dose Pills," *Family Planning Perspectives* 16/5 (1984): 237–38.

91. Sybil Shainwald, National Women's Health Network and attorney for Dalkon Shield plaintiffs, personal communication with author, June 21, 1986.

Chapter 3

1. "Two Apostles of Control," *Life,* April 17, 1970, 32–37.

2. Alan F. Guttmacher, *Birth Control and Love: The Complete Guide to Contraception and Fertility,* 2d rev. ed. (London: Macmillan, 1969), 118.

3. *Population Research: Mankind's Great Need* (Washington: Population Crisis Committee, 1971).

4. Betsy Hartmann, *Reproductive Rights and Wrongs: The Global Politics of Population Control and Contraceptive Choice* (New York: Harper and Row, 1987), 273, 274.

5. Garrett Hardin, *Birth Control* (New York: Pegasus, 1970), 126, 127.

6. Ibid., 126.

7. Guttmacher, *Birth Control and Love*, 43.

8. Ibid., 49.

9. U.S. Food and Drug Administration, Advisory Committee on Obstetrics and Gynecology, *Report on Intrauterine Contraceptive Devices* (1968 [Document No. 29-137 0-68-3]), 1.

10. Hugh J. Davis, *Intrauterine Devices for Contraception: The IUD* (Baltimore: Williams and Wilkins, 1971), 22–23.

11. Ibid., 77.

12. U.S. FDA, *Report on Intrauterine Contraceptive Devices*, 32.

13. Clive Wood, *Intrauterine Devices* (London: Butterworth, 1971), 49, 87, 125.

14. Ibid., 86.

15. Boston Women's Health Collective, *Our Bodies, Ourselves* (New York: Simon and Schuster, 1973).

16. Bruce V. Stadel and Sarah Schlesselman, "Extent of Surgery for Pelvic Inflammatory Disease in Relation to Duration of Intrauterine Device Use," *Obstetrics and Gynecology* 63 (1984): 177; L. D. Gruer, K. E. Collingsham, and C. W. Edwards, "Pneumococcal Peritonitis Associated with an IUD," *The Lancet*, September 17, 1983, 677; Mary C. Jones et al., "The Prevalence of Actinomycetis-like Organisms Found in Cervicovaginal Smears of 300 IUD Wearers," *Acta Cytologica* 23 (1979): 283.

17. Paul K. O'Brien, "Abdominal and Endometrial Actinomycosis Associated with an Intrauterine Device," *Canadian Medical Association Journal* 112 (1975): 596, 597.

18. Waldemar A. Schmidt, "IUDs, Inflammation, and Infection: Assessment after Two Decades of IUD Use," *Human Pathology* 13 (1982): 879.

19. Julian Elias, "Intra-Uterine Contraceptive Devices," *The Practitioner* 229 (1985): 431–36.

20. Schmidt, "IUDs, Inflammation, and Infection," 879.

21. Wood, *Intrauterine Devices*, 97–98.

22. Mahmood Yoonessi et al., "Association of Actinomyces and Intrauterine Contraceptive Devices," *Journal of Reproductive Medicine* 30 (1985): 51; Michael J. Colin and Gerald Weissman, "Disseminated Gonococcal Infection and Tenosynovitis from an Asymptomatically Infected Intrauterine Contraceptive Device," *New England Journal of Medicine* 294 (1976): 598–99.

23. Colin and Weissman, "Disseminated Gonococcal Infection," 598–99.

24. Timothy J. Herbert and P. P. Mortimer, "Recurrent Pneumonococcal Peritonitis Associated with an Intra-uterine Contraceptive Device," *British Journal of Surgery* 61 (1974): 901–2; Ira M. Golditch and James E. Huston, "Serious Pelvic Infections Associated with Intrauterine Contraceptive Device," *International Journal of Fertility* 18 (1973): 158; P. A. Smith et al., "Deaths Associated with Intrauterine Contraceptive Devices in the United Kingdom between 1973 and 1983," *British Medical Journal* 287 (1983): 1537–38; Schmidt, "IUDs, Inflammation, and Infection," 878–81.

25. Schmidt, "IUDs, Inflammation, and Infection," 878; E. Persson et al., "Actinomyces Israelii in the Genital Tract of Women with and without Intra-uterine Contraceptive Devices," *Acta Obstetricia Gynecologica Scandinavica* 62 (1983): 563; John Kelly and Janice Aaron, "Pelvic Actinomycosis and Usage of Intrauterine Contraceptive Devices," *Yale Journal of Biology and Medicine* 55 (1982): 460; Persson et al., "Actinomyces Israelii," 563; William Bonnez et al., "Actinomyces Naeslundii as an Agent of Pelvic Actinomycosis in the Presence of an Intrauterine Device," *Journal of Clinical Microbiology* 21 (1985): 273; Kelly and Aaron, "Pelvic Actinomycosis," 460; E. Persson and K. Holmberg, "Genital Colonization by Actinomyces Israelii and Serologic Immune Response to the Bacterium after Five Years Use of the Same Copper Intra-Uterine Device," *Acta Obstetricia Gynecologica Scandinavica* 63 (1984): 205.

26. Theodore C. Nagel, "Intrauterine Contraceptive Devices: Complications Associated with Their Use," *Postgraduate Medicine* 73 (1983): 163; Stadel and Schlesselman, "Extent of Surgery," 176.

27. Susanne Morgan, *Coping with Hysterectomy: Your Own Choice, Your Own Solutions* (New York: Dial, 1982), 49–52, "Rates of Unnecessary Surgery"; Yoonessi et al., "Actinomyces and Intrauterine Contraceptive Devices," 52; Diane Scully, *Men Who Control Women's Health: The Miseducation of Obstetrician-Gynecologists* (Boston: Houghton Mifflin, 1980), 142; Boston Women's Health Collective, *The New Our Bodies, Ourselves* (New York: Simon and Schuster, 1984), 511; Hysterectomy and Educational Resources and Services (HERS), suggested reading list (write 501 Woodbrook Lane, Philadelphia, PA 19119); L. Zussman et al., "Sexual Response after Hysterectomy-Oophorectomy: Recent Studies and Reconsideration of Psychogenesis," *American Journal of Obstetrics and Gynecology* 140 (1981): 725–29.

28. Simon Henderson, "Pelvic Actinomycosis Associated with an Intrauterine Device," *Obstetrics and Gynecology* 41 (1973): 726–32.

29. R. Snowden and B. Pearson, "Pelvic Infection: A Comparison of the Dalkon Shield and Three Other Intrauterine Devices," *British Medical Journal* 288 (1984): 1571; David W. Kaufman et al., "The Effects of Different Types of Intrauterine Devices on the Risk of Pelvic Inflammatory Disease," *Journal of the American Medical Association* 250 (1983): 759.

30. Schmidt, "IUDs, Inflammation, and Infection," 878, 879; Susan Perry and Jim Dawson, *Nightmare: Women and the Dalkon Shield* (New York: Macmillan, 1985), 50.

31. Stadel and Schlesselman, "Extent of Surgery," 177; Mary Pollock, "Letting Intrauterine Devices Lie," *British Medical Journal* 285 (1982): 1049.

32. Howard Ory and the Women's Health Study, "Ectopic Pregnancy and Intrauterine Contraceptive Devices: New Perspectives," *Obstetrics and Gynecology* 57 (1981): 143; Steven H. Eisinger, "Second-trimester Spontaneous Abortion, the IUD, and Infection," *American Journal of Obstetrics and Gynecology* 124 (1976): 393–97; Willard Cates, Jr., et al., "The Intrauterine Device and Deaths from Spontaneous Abortion," *New England Journal of Medicine* 295 (1976): 1155; H. Robert Misenhimer and Rafael Garcia-Bunuel, "Failure of an Intrauterine Contraceptive Device and Fungal Infection in the Fetus," *Obstetrics and Gynecology* 34 (1969): 368–72; "A. H. Robins Co. Pays $1.4 Million to Settle Contraceptive Suit," *Wall Street Journal*, March 17, 1980, 19; William J. Ledger and Frank J. Schrader, "Death from Septicemia Following Insertion of an Intrauterine Device: Report of a Case," *Obstetrics and Gynecology* 31 (1968): 845–48; R. A. Sparks, letter, *The Lancet*, April 28,

1984, 957; R. D. Patchell, "Rectouterine Fistula Associated with the Cu-7 Intrauterine Contraceptive Device," *American Journal of Obstetrics and Gynecology* 126 (1976): 292–93; P. K. Heinonen, M. Merikari, and J. Paavonen, "Uterine Perforation by Copper Intrauterine Device," *European Journal of Obstetrics, Gynecology, and Reproductive Medicine* 17 (1984): 260; Joseph D'Amico and Robert Israel, "Bowel Obstruction and Perforation with an Inter-peritoneal Loop Intrauterine Contraceptive Device," *American Journal of Obstetrics and Gynecology* 129 (1977): 461–62; Eberhard Neutz, Arthur Silber, and Vincent J. Meredino, "Dalkon Shield Perforation of the Uterus and Urinary Bladder with Calculus Formation: Case Report," *American Journal of Obstetrics and Gynecology* 130 (1978): 848–49; R. Mark Kirk, "Ureteral Obstruction Complicating the IUD," *Journal of the American Medical Association* 215 (1971): 1156; J. A. Goldman et al., "Case Report: IUD Appendicitis," *European Journal of Obstetrics, Gynecology, and Reproductive Medicine* 15 (1983): 181–83; William K. Blenkinsopp and Patricia Chapman, "Prevalence of Cervical Neoplasia and Infection in Women Using Intrauterine Contraceptive Devices," *Journal of Reproductive Medicine* 27 (1982): 712; Thomas W. McElin, "Severe Peritonitis and the IUD," *American Journal of Obstetrics and Gynecology* 113 (1972): 570; Drorith Hochner-Celnikier et al., "Pelvic Abscess Associated with a Lippes Loop: An Unusual Case," *Journal of Reproductive Medicine* 28 (1983): 543.

33. U.S. FDA, *Report on Intrauterine Contraceptive Devices*, 6; Ory and the Women's Health Study, "Ectopic Pregnancy," 143.

34. R. J. Beerthuizen et al., "IUD and Salpingitis: A Prospective Study of Patho-morphological Changes in the Oviducts of IUD Users," *European Journal of Obstetrics, Gynecology, and Reproductive Biology* 13 (1982): 31–41; Anne Lone Wollen, Per R. Flood, Roar Sandvei, and Johan A. Steier, "Morphological Changes in Tubal Mucosa Associated with the Use of Intrauterine Contraceptive Devices," *British Journal of Obstetrics and Gynecology* 91 (1984): 1123–28.

35. P. A. Smith et al., "Deaths Associated with Intrauterine Contraceptive Devices," 1537–38.

36. D. F. Hawkins, "Intrauterine Contraception," *The Practitioner* 205 (1970): 20.

37. Scully, *Men Who Control Women's Health*, 92.

38. Wood, *Intrauterine Devices*, 90.

39. Sylvia Wasserthal-Smoller et al., "Contraceptive Practices of Wives of Obstetricians," *American Journal of Obstetrics and Gynecology* 117 (1973): 709–15; Charles F. Westoff, "The Modernization of U.S. Contraceptive Practice," *Family Planning Perspectives* 4/3 (1972): 9–12.

Chapter 4

1. Robert W. Kistner, "What 'the Pill' Does to Husbands," *Ladies' Home Journal,* January 1969, 66.

2. "Gossypol Prospects," *The Lancet,* May 19, 1984, 1108–9; "Gossypol," *Journal of the American Medical Association* 252 (1984): 1102–3.

3. Bette Weinstein, "Birth Control Pill for Men," *McCall's,* July 1974, 34–35.

4. M. M. Kapur et al., "Copper Intravas Device (IVD) and Male Contraception," *Contraception* 29 (1984): 45–54.

5. Alan F. Guttmacher, *Birth Control and Love: The Complete Guide to Contraception and Fertility,* 2d rev. ed. (London: Macmillan, 1969), 14.

6. Garrett Hardin, *Birth Control* (New York: Pegasus, 1970), 72–73.

7. Hugh J. Davis, *Intrauterine Devices for Contraception: The IUD* (Baltimore: Williams and Wilkins, 1971), 19.

8. Barbara Seaman, "Tell Me Doctor: 'Why Did Birth Control Fail Me?'" *Ladies' Home Journal*, November 1965, 167.

9. Ian S. Fraser and Robert P. S. Jansen, "Why Do Inadvertent Pregnancies Occur in Oral Contraceptive Users? Effectiveness of Oral Contraceptive Regimens and Interfering Factors," *Contraception* 27 (1983): 531–51.

10. Shere Hite, *The Hite Report: A Nationwide Study of Female Sexuality*, rev. ed. (New York: Dell, 1981). Also see *The Hite Report on Male Sexuality: How Men Feel about Love, Sex, and Relationships* (New York: Ballantine, 1982).

11. Boston Women's Health Collective, *The New Our Bodies, Ourselves* (New York: Simon and Schuster, 1984), 237.

12. Grantly Dick-Read, *Childbirth without Fear*, 4th rev. ed. (New York: Harper and Row, 1978 [originally published 1949]).

13. Richard M. Frank and Christopher Tietze, "Acceptance of an Oral Contraceptive Program in a Large Metropolitan Area," *American Journal of Obstetrics and Gynecology* 93 (1965): 122–27.

14. "Birth Control Pills: An Up-to-Date Report," *Good Housekeeping*, September 1965, 160.

15. Francis J. Kane, Jr., "Psychiatric Reactions to Oral Contraceptives," *American Journal of Obstetrics and Gynecology* 102 (1968): 1059.

16. Ibid., 1061.

17. Ibid., 1062.

18. Naomi M. Morris and J. Richard Udry, "Depression of Physical Activity by Contraceptive Pills," *American Journal of Obstetrics and Gynecology* 104 (1969): 1014.

19. A. W. Diddle, William H. Gardner, and Perry J. Williamson, "Oral Contraceptive Medications and Headache," *American Journal of Obstetrics and Gynecology* 105 (1969): 509.

20. "FDA Unit Urges Ban on A. H. Robins IUD Continue until Study," *Wall Street Journal*, August 26, 1974, 14.

21. "A. H. Robins to Collect Unused IUDs in U.S., Slates Modification," *Wall Street Journal*, January 21, 1975, 12; "Maker of Dalkon Shield Urges Removal of Devices from Women Having Them," *Wall Street Journal*, September 26, 1980, 12.

Chapter 5

1. U.S. Congress, House, Committee on Population, *The Depo-Provera Debate* (95th Cong., 2d sess., 1978): 189 (breast cancer); 201 (stroke); 83–86 (amenorrhea); 79 (headaches); 200 (weight gain); 197 (permanent infertility); 114 (loss of libido); 182 (clitoral hypertrophy in the fetus); 74 (cardiac defects and limb reduction in the fetus).

2. Ibid., 155.

3. Ibid., 46.

4. Ibid., 23, 53.

5. Ibid., 168.

6. Ibid., 19.

7. Ibid., 11, 14, 25, 83, 86.

8. Ibid., 11.

9. Ibid., 27.

10. National Women's Health Network, *Depoprovera* (Washington: NWHN, 1985).

11. "Hormonal Contraceptives: Long-Acting Methods," *Population Reports*, ser. K, no. 3 (vol. 15/1 [Baltimore: Johns Hopkins University, Population Information Program, 1987]), K58–K84; Betsy Hartmann, *Reproductive Rights and Wrongs: The Global Politics of Population Control and Contraceptive Choice* (New York: Harper and Row, 1987), 170–71, 196–200; "Long-Acting Progestins—Promise and Prospects," *Population Reports*, ser. K, no. 2 (vol. 11/2 [Baltimore: Johns Hopkins University, Population Information Program, 1983]), K17–K55.

12. Michael Brody, "When Products Turn into Liabilities," *Fortune*, March 3, 1986, 20; "IUDs—A New Look," *Population Reports*, ser. B, no. 5 (vol. 16/1 [Baltimore: Johns Hopkins University, Population Information Program, 1988]), 2–31.

13. "IUDs—A New Look," 3.

14. Ibid., 8.

15. Ellen Sweet, "A Failed 'Revolution,' " *Ms.*, March 1988, 75.

16. Ibid.

17. Ibid., 77–78.

18. Ibid., 76.

19. Doris Haire, *How the FDA Determines the "Safety" of Drugs—Just How Safe Is "Safe"? A Report Released to the Congress of the United States* (Washington: National Women's Health Network, 1984), 1.

Chapter 6

1. See Mark Dowie, "The Corporate Crime of the Century," *Mother Jones*, November 1979.

2. Betsy Hartmann, *Reproductive Rights and Wrongs: The Global Politics of Contraceptive Choice* (New York: Harper and Row, 1987).

3. Gena Corea, *The Mother Machine: Reproductive Technologies from Artificial Insemination to Artificial Wombs* (New York: Harper and Row, 1985), 287. Also see Corea's *The Hidden Malpractice: How American Medicine Mistreats Women*, updated ed. (New York: Harper and Row, 1985).

4. Andrea Dworkin, *Intercourse* (New York: Free Press, 1987), 152, 158.

5. Ibid., 128–29, 133.

6. Barbara Ehrenreich, *The Hearts of Men* (New York: Anchor, 1984), 11–13; Barbara Ehrenreich and Dierdre English, *For Her Own Good: 150 Years of the Experts' Advice to Women* (Garden City, N.Y.: Anchor, 1979), 196–210, 237–41, 318–24.

7. Germaine Greer, *Sex and Destiny: The Politics of Human Fertility* (New York: Harper and Row, 1984), esp. 286–88.

8. Betty Friedan, *The Second Stage* (New York: Summit, 1981), 41; Judith Stacey, "Are Feminists Afraid to Leave Home? The Challenge of Conservative Pro-family Feminism," in *What Is Feminism? A Re-examination*, ed. Juliet Mitchell and Ann Oakley (New York: Pantheon, 1986), 213, 221.

9. Linda Kerber, "Separate Spheres, Female Worlds, Woman's Place: The Rhetoric of Women's History," *Journal of American History* 75 (1988): 39.

10. Heidi Hartmann, "Changes in Women's Economic and Family Roles in Post–World War II United States," in *Women, Households and the Economy*, ed. Lourdes Beneira and Catherine A. Stimpson (New Brunswick: Rutgers University Press, 1987), 33.

11. Ibid., 36, 41.

12. Ibid., 41.

13. Ibid., 45.

14. Jerzy Berent, "Family Size Preference in Europe and U.S.A.: Ultimate Expected Number of Children," *World Fertility Surveys* (1983): 27, table 16.

15. Beverly Wildung Harrison, *Our Right to Choose: Toward a New Ethic of Abortion* (Boston: Beacon, 1983), 45.

16. Mina Davis Caulfield, "Sexuality in Human Evolution: What Is 'Natural' in Sex?" *Feminist Studies* 11 (1985): 353.

Bibliography

"A. H. Robins Co. Plans to Continue Marketing Its Dalkon Shield IUD." *Wall Street Journal*, May 29, 1974, 8.

"A. H. Robins to Collect Unused IUDs in U.S., Slates Modification." *Wall Street Journal*, January 21, 1975, 12.

"A. H. Robins Will Stop Sale of Dalkon Shield, Pending Safety Study." *Wall Street Journal*, May 30, 1974, 36.

"A. H. Robins Wins Clearance from FDA to Resume IUD Sale." *Wall Street Journal*, December 23, 1974, 7.

Abdulla, K. A., Sawsan I. Elwan, H. S. Salem, and M. M. Shaahan. "Effect of Early Postpartum Use of the Contraceptive Implants, Norplant, on the Serum Levels of Immunoglobulins of the Mothers and Their Breastfed Infants." *Contraception* 32 (1985): 261–66.

Abraham, A. Andrew. "Herpesvirus Hominis Endometritis in a Young Woman Wearing an Intrauterine Contraceptive." *American Journal of Obstetrics and Gynecology* 131 (1978): 340–42.

Acker, David, Frank H. Boehm, Denny E. Askew, and Howard Rothman. "Electrocardiogram Changes with Intrauterine Contraceptive Device Insertion." *American Journal of Obstetrics and Gynecology* 115 (1973): 458–61.

"Actinomyces-like Organisms and IUD Use Linked But Clinical Importance of the Finding Is Unclear." *Family Planning Perspectives* 14/1 (1982): 34–35.

Agnew, H. Wayne, and Jack A. Pritchard. "Abortion and Bacterial Shock Induced with an Intrauterine Contraceptive Device: Report of a Case." *Obstetrics and Gynecology* 28 (1966): 332–34.

Aldridge, Leslie. "Why They Quit the Pill." *McCall's*, November 1968.

Allen, E. Stewart, and Willis E. Brown. "An Evaluation of Local Reaction to an Intrauterine Contraceptive Device: The Grafenberg Ring" *Obstetrics and Gynecology* 23 (1964): 638–39.

"Are IUDs *Really* Safe?" *Good Housekeeping*, January 1975, 127.

Aronson, H. Benzion, Florella Magora, and J. G. Schenker. "Effect of Oral Contraceptives on Blood Viscosity." *American Journal of Obstetrics and Gynecology* 110 (1971): 997–1001.

Athari, Terry A., and Cesar Pizarro. "Perforation of the Large Bowel by a Dalkon Shield Intrauterine Device." *Journal of Reproductive Medicine* 17 (1976): 331–32.

"Bacterial Endocarditis after Insertion of Intrauterine Contraceptive Device." *British Medical Journal*, July 12, 1975, 76–77.

Baehler, Elizabeth A., William P. Dillon, Diane M. Dryja, and Erwin Neter. "The Effects of Prolonged Retention of Diaphragms on Colonization by Staphylococcus Aureus of the Lower Genital Tract." *Fertility and Sterility* 39 (1983): 162–66.

"Ban on Robins' IUD Becomes More Likely after New U.S. Study." *Wall Street Journal*, July 5, 1974, 15.

Bank, Harvey, Marsha MacDonald, and Susan Wiechert. "Fluid Migration through the Tail of the Dalkon Shield Intrauterine Device." *Contraception* 29 (1984): 65–75.

Banks, Joseph Ambrose. *Prosperity and Parenthood: A Study of Family Planning among the Victorian Middle Classes.* London: Routledge and Kegan Paul, 1954.

Banks, Joseph Ambrose, and Olive Banks. *Feminism and Family Planning in Victorian England.* New York: Schocken, 1974.

Beecham, Jackson B., John Van S. Maech, and Philip B. Mead. "Severe Pelvic Sepsis and the Majzlin Spring." *Obstetrics and Gynecology* 43 (1974): 159.

Beerthuizen, R. J., J.A.M. Van Wijck, T.K.A.B. Eskes, A.H.M. Vermeulen, and G. P. Vooijs. "IUD and Salpingitis: A Prospective Study of Pathomorphological Changes in the Oviducts of IUD-Users." *European Journal of Obstetrics, Gynecology, and Reproductive Biology* 13 (1982): 31–41.

Behrman, S. J., and William Burchfield. "The Intrauterine Contraceptive Device and Myometrial Activity." *American Journal of Obstetrics and Gynecology* 100 (1968): 194–202.

Beljadj, Hedia, Irving Sivin, Solidad Diaz, Margarita Panez, Ana-Sofia Tejada, Vivian Brache, Francisco Alvarez, Donna Shoupe, Marlene Breaux, D. R. Mishell, Jr., Terry McCarthy, and Veronica Yo. "Recovery of Fertility after Use of the Levonorgestril 20 nicg/d or Copper T 380 Ag Intrauterine Device." *Contraception* 34 (1986): 261–67.

Belsey, Elizabeth M., David Machin, and Catherine d'Arcangues. "The Analysis of Vaginal Bleeding Patterns Induced by Fertility Regulating Methods." *Contraception* 34 (1986): 253–61.

Beneira, Lourdes, and Catherine A. Stimpson, eds. *Women, Households and the Economy.* New Brunswick: Rutgers University Press, 1987.

Bengtson, Lars Philip, and Atef H. Moawad. "The Effect of the Lippes Loop on Human Myometrial Activity." *American Journal of Obstetrics and Gynecology* 98 (1967): 957–65.

Benson, Michael D., and Robert W. Rebar. "Relationship of Migraine Headache and Stroke to Oral Contraceptive Use." *Journal of Reproductive Medicine* 31 (1986): 1082–88.

Berent, Jerzy. "Family Size Preference in Europe and U.S.A.: Ultimate Expected Number of Children." *World Fertility Surveys* (1983): 27.

Berkman, Joyce Avrech. "History of Contraceptive Advocacy." In *Birth Control and Controlling Birth: Woman-Centered Perspectives,* ed. Helen B. Holmes, Betty B. Hoskins, and Michael Gross, 37–46. Clifton, N.J.: Humana, 1980.

Berlin, Elois Ann. "Aspects of Fertility Regulation among the Aguaruna Jivaro of Peru." In *Women's Medicine,* ed. Lucile F. Newman, 125–46. New Brunswick: Rutgers University Press, 1985.

Berman, Donald H. *The Role of Law in Population Planning: Working Paper and Proceedings of the Sixteenth Hammarskjold Forum.* New York: Oceana, 1972.

Bernard, R. P. "Factors Governing IUD Performance." *American Journal of Public Health* 61 (1971): 559–67.

Bernstein, Gerald S. "Conventional Methods of Contraception: Condom, Diaphragm, and Vaginal Foam." *Clinical Obstetrics and Gynecology* 17 (1974): 21–23.

Best, Winfield. "Something New in Birth Control: A Report on the Remarkably Effective IUCD's—The Latest Development in Family-Limitation Techniques." *Reader's Digest,* April 1965, 79–82. (Condensed from *McCall's*)

Beyer, George, and S. J. Behrman. "Myometrial Activity and the IUCD: Ill Effect of Contraceptive Pills." *American Journal of Obstetrics and Gynecology* 106 (1970): 87–92.

Birdsall, Nancy, and Lauren A. Chester. "Contraception and the Status of Women: What Is the Link?" *Family Planning Perspectives* 19/1 (1987): 14–18.

Birnberg, Charles, and Michael S. Burnhill. "Whither the IUD? The Present and Future of Intrauterine Contraceptives." *Obstetrics and Gynecology* 31 (1968): 861–65.

"Birth Control: Is Male Contraception the Answer?" *Good Housekeeping,* April 1969, 201–03.

"Birth Control: A Summary and Chart of Current Contraceptive Measures." *Good Housekeeping,* February 1974, 176–77.

"Birth Control: An Up-to-Date Summary of Contraceptive Methods." *Good Housekeeping,* January 1967, 144–45.

Birth Control and Morality in Nineteenth Century America. New York: Arno Press, 1972.

"The Birth Control Method That May Replace 'the Pill.'" *Good Housekeeping,* April 1966, 177–79.

"Birth Control Pills: An Up-to-Date Report." *Good Housekeeping,* September 1965, 159–61.

Black, C., and V. P. Houghton. "A User Acceptability Study of Vaginal Spermicides in Combination with Barrier Methods or an IUCD." *Contraception* 28 (1983): 103–10.

Blenkinsopp, William K., and Patricia Chapman. "Prevalence of Cervical Neoplasia and Infection in Women Using Intrauterine Contraceptive Devices." *Journal of Reproductive Medicine* 27 (1982): 709–13.

Blum, Sam. "The Pill." *Redbook,* January 1966.

Bonnez, William, Gary Lattimer, Navaratnasingam A. C. Mohanraj, and Theodore H. Johnson. "Actinomyces Naeslundii as an Agent of Pelvic Actinomycosis in the Presence of an Intrauterine Device." *Journal of Clinical Microbiology* 21 (1985): 273–75.

Boston Women's Health Collective. *The New Our Bodies, Ourselves.* New York: Simon and Schuster, 1984.

———. *Our Bodies, Ourselves: A Book by and for Women.* New York: Simon and Schuster, 1973.

Bowman, James A., Jr. "The Effect of Norethindrone-mestranol on Cervical Mucus." *American Journal of Obstetrics and Gynecology* 102 (1968): 1039–40.

Boyd, J. D., and K. F. Rawlinson. "Third-Trimester Uterine Sepsis Associated with Shield-Type Intrauterine Device." *The Lancet,* April 5, 1975, 813.

Bozza, Anthony T., and S. Theodore Horwitz. "Ovarian Pregnancy with an Intrauterine Contraceptive Device in Situ: A Case Report." *American Journal of Obstetrics and Gynecology* 117 (1973): 785–86.

"Breakthrough in Birth Control." *Reader's Digest,* January 1966, 61–64. (Condensed from *U.S. News and World Report*)

Breed, W. G. "The Efficiency of the Dalkon Shield." *Medical Journal of Australia,* June 8, 1974, 943.

Breen, James L. "A 21 Year Survey of 654 Ectopic Pregnancies." *American Journal of Obstetrics and Gynecology* 106 (1970): 1004–19.

Bremmer, William J., and David M. de Kretser. "Contraceptive for Males." *SIGNS: Journal of Women in Culture and Society* 1 (1975): 387–96.

———. "The Prospects for New, Reversible Male Contraceptives." *New England Journal of Medicine* 295 (1976): 111–17.

Brenner, Paul F., Donna L. Cooper, and Daniel R. Michell, Jr. "Clinical Study of a Progesterone-Releasing Intrauterine Contraceptive Device." *American Journal of Obstetrics and Gynecology* 121 (1975): 704–06.

Brenner, Richard W., and Samuel W. Gehring II. "Pelvic Actinomycosis in the Presence of an Endocervical Contraceptive Device: Report of a Case." *Obstetrics and Gynecology* 29 (1967): 71–73.

Brody, Eugene B. "Everyday Knowledge of Jamaican Women." In *Women's Medicine*, ed. Lucile F. Newman, 161–78. New Brunswick: Rutgers University Press, 1985.

Brody, Michael. "When Products Turn into Liabilities." *Fortune*, March 3, 1986.

Brooks, Philip G., George Berci, Allen Lawrence, Philip Slipyan, and Maclyn E. Wade. "Removal of Intra-abdominal Intrauterine Contraceptive Devices through a Peritoneoscope with the Use of Intraoperative Fluoroscopy to Aid Localization." *American Journal of Obstetrics and Gynecology* 113 (1972): 104–06.

Browner, C. H. "Traditional Techniques for Diagnosis, Treatment and Control of Pregnancy in Cali, Colombia." In *Women's Medicine*, ed. Lucile F. Newman, 99–124. New Brunswick: Rutgers University Press, 1985.

Bruce, J., and S. B. Schaerer. *Contraceptives and Common Sense: Conventional Methods Reconsidered.* New York: Population Council, 1979.

Brueschke, Erich E., James R. Wingfield, Marvin Burns, and Lourens J. D. Zaneveld. "Development of a Reversible Vas Deferens Occlusive Device. II. Effect of Bilateral and Unilateral Vasectomy on Semen Characteristics in the Dog." *Fertility and Sterility* 25 (1974): 673–86.

Brueschke, Erich E., Marvin Burns, John H. Maness, James R. Wingfield, Kenneth Mayerhofer, and Lourens J. D. Zaneveld. "Development of a Reversible Vas Deferens Occlusive Device. I. Anatomical Size of the Human and Dog Vas Deferens." *Fertility and Sterility* 25 (1974): 659–72.

Brueschke, Erich E., Lourens J. D. Zaneveld, Richard Rodzen, and Dennis Berns. "Development of a Reversible Vas Deferens Occlusive Device. III. Morphology of the Human and Dog Vas Deferens: A Study with the Scanning Electron Microscope." *Fertility and Sterility* 25 (1974): 687–702.

Buckingham, M. S., R. A. Sparks, Peter J. Watt, and Max Elstein. "Pelvic Infection and Intrauterine Devices." *British Medical Journal*, October 16, 1976, 942–43.

Buhler, M., and E. Papiernik. "Successive Pregnancies in Women Fitted with Intrauterine Devices Who Take Anti-inflammatory Drugs." *The Lancet*, February 26, 1983, 483.

Burkman, Ronald T., and the Women's Health Study. "Association between Intrauterine Device and Pelvic Inflammatory Disease." *Obstetrics and Gynecology* 57 (1981): 269–75.

Burnhill, Michael S. "Perforation of Uterus in Association with IUD." *Obstetrics and Gynecology* 29 (1967): 731.

Burnhill, Michael S., and Charles H. Birnberg. "Contraception with an Intrauterine Bow Inserted Immediately Post Partum: An Interim Report." *Obstetrics and Gynecology* 28 (1966): 329–30.

————. "Uterine Perforation with Intrauterine Contraceptive Devices: Review of the Literature and Cases Reported to the National Committee on Maternal Health." *American Journal of Obstetrics and Gynecology* 98 (1967): 135–39.

Burry, Kenneth A., and Martin L. Pernoll. "The Fragmented Intrauterine Device: An Unusual Complication of a Lippes Loop." *Fertility and Sterility* 29 (1978): 218–19.

Cade, Toni. "The Pill: Genocide or Liberation?" In *The Black Woman: An Anthology,* ed. Toni Cade, 162–69. New York: Mentor, 1970.

Calderone, Mary Steicher, ed. *Manual of Family Planning and Contraceptive Practice.* Baltimore: Williams and Wilkins, 1970.

Cassell, Carol. *Swept Away: Why Women Confuse Love and Sex . . . and How They Can Have Both.* New York: Bantam, 1984.

Cates, Willard, Jr., Howard W. Ory, Roger W. Rochat, and Carl W. Tyler, Jr. "The Intrauterine Device and Deaths from Spontaneous Abortion." *New England Journal of Medicine* 295 (1976): 1155–59.

Caulfield, Mina Davis. "Sexuality in Human Evolution: What Is 'Natural' in Sex?" *Feminist Studies* 11 (1985).

Cederqvist, Lars L., and Fritz Fuchs. "Cervical Perforation by the Copper T Intrauterine Contraceptive Device." *American Journal of Obstetrics and Gynecology* 119 (1974): 854–55.

Cederqvist, Lars L., Zoltan S. Saary, and Soannis A. Zervondakis. "Translocation of the Dalkon Shield into the Broad Ligament." *Obstetrics and Gynecology* 46 (1975): 239–42.

"Cervical Cap Study Finds Eight Pregnancies Per 100 Users Per Year, Continuation Rate of 67 Percent." *Family Planning Perspectives* 14/4 (1982): 215–16.

Chadwick, John M. "The Dalkon Shield Contraceptive Device for General Practice." *Medical Journal of Australia,* October 4, 1975, 565–66.

Chapel, Thomas A. "Oral Contraceptives and Exacerbation of Lupus Erythematosus." *American Journal of Obstetrics and Gynecology* 110 (1971): 366–69.

Chaudhuri, G. "Inhibition by Aspirin and Indomethacin of Uterine Hypertrophy Induced by an IUD." *Journal of Reproduction and Fertility* 43 (1975): 77–81.

Chi, I. Cheng, Leonard Laufe, and Susan Rogers. "IUD-Associated Hospitalization in Less Developed Countries." *American Journal of Public Health* 74 (1984): 353–57.

Chi, I. Cheng, Lynne R. Wilkins, Albert J. Siemens, and Jack Lippes. "Syncope and Other Vascular Reactions at Interval Insertion of Lippes Loop D—Who Is Most Vulnerable?" *Contraception* 33 (1986): 179–87.

Child, Marion. "Birth Control: Why Shouldn't Your Husband Take a Pill?" *Redbook,* February 1973, 96–97.

Chow, Anthony W., Kay L. Malkasian, John R. Marshall, and Lucien B. Guze. "The Bacteriology of Acute Pelvic Inflammatory Disease: Value of Cul-de-sac Cultures and Relative Importance of Gonococci and Other Aerobic and Anaerobic Bacteria." *American Journal of Obstetrics and Gynecology* 122 (1975): 876–79.

Christian, C. D. "Maternal Deaths Associated with an Intrauterine Device." *American Journal of Obstetrics and Gynecology* 119 (1974): 441–44.

Chung, Arthur F., and Stanley J. Burnbaum. "Pseudoectopic Intrauterine Contraceptive Device (A Case Report)." *American Journal of Obstetrics and Gynecology* 114 (1972): 272–73.

Claman, A. David. "A Trial of a One Dose a Month Oral Contraceptive." *American Journal of Obstetrics and Gynecology* 107 (1970): 461–64.

Colin, Michael J., and Gerald Weissman. "Disseminated Gonococcal Infection and Tenosynovitis from an Asymptomatically Infected Intrauterine Contraceptive Device." *New England Journal of Medicine* 294 (1976): 598–99.

Collins, J. A., P. G. Gillett, S. A. Perlin, J. A. Embil, I. Zayid, G. Richards, and M. E. Kirk. "Microbiological and Histological Findings in the Fallopian Tubes of Women Using Various Contraceptive Methods." *Contraception* 30 (1984): 457–66.

Connell, Elizabeth B. "The Pill in Perspective." *Reader's Digest,* October 1970, 118–21.

———. "The Search for the Ideal Contraceptive." *Redbook,* January 1984.

"Contraception: Comparing the Options." *FDA Consumer,* July–August 1977, 7–13.

"Contraceptive Claims Scaled Down." *FDA Consumer,* May 1980, 3.

"Contraceptive Pill: FDA Writes Another Warning." *Science News* 97 (1970): 599.

"Contraceptives: Further Evidence on Clots." *Science News* 95 (1969): 644, col. 2.

"Contraceptive Warning: FDA Goes to the Consumer." *Science News* 97 (1970): 266.

Cordero, Jose F., and Peter M. Layde. "Vaginal Spermicides, Chromosomal Abnormalities and Limb Reduction Defects." *International Family Planning Perspectives* 9 (1983): 15–18.

Corea, Gena. *The Hidden Malpractice: How American Medicine Mistreats Women.* Updated ed. New York: Harper and Row, 1985.

———. *The Mother Machine: Reproductive Technologies from Artificial Insemination to Artificial Wombs.* New York: Harper and Row, 1985.

"Crackdown." *Newsweek,* November 2, 1970, 100.

Craig, John M. "The Pathology of Birth Control." *Archives of Pathology* 99 (1975): 233–36.

Craig, Sue, and Sue Hepburn. "The Effectiveness of Barrier Methods of Contraception with and without Spermicide." *Contraception* 26 (1982): 347–59.

Croxatto, Horatio. "A Mode of Action of IUDs." *Fertility and Sterility* 39 (1983): 114.

"Cryosurgery Recommended for Cervical Eversion." *Journal of the American Medical Association* 216 (1971): 601.

"Cu-7 IUD Can Be Used up to Four Years with Low Pregnancy Rates." *Family Planning Perspectives* 14/1 (1982): 35–36.

Culliford, Alfred T., Matthew N. Harris, Robert F. Porges, Peter H. Berczeller, Edward L. Amorosi, and W. Robson N. Grier. "Streptococcal Peritonitis in a Patient with Hodgkin's Disease and an Intrauterine Contraceptive Device." *American Journal of Obstetrics and Gynecology* 117 (1973): 288–89.

"Cures That Can Kill." *Newsweek,* November 2, 1970, 100.

"Dalkon IUD Won't Be Returned to Market." *FDA Consumer,* September 1975, 25.

"The Dalkon Shield." *FDA Consumer,* February 1975, 21.

"The Dalkon Shield Contraceptive Device in General Practice." *Medical Journal of Australia,* October 4, 1975, 565–66.

"The Dalkon Shield Intrauterine Device." *Medical Letter on Drugs and Therapeutics* 14 (1971): 97–98.

"Dalkon Shield Suits against Robins Rise, SEC Report Shows." *Wall Street Journal,* January 21, 1975, 12.

"Dalkon Shield Warning." *FDA Consumer,* July–August 1983, 2.

Daly, Mary. *Gyn/Ecology: The Metaethics of Radical Feminism.* Boston: Beacon, 1978.

D'Amico, Joseph, and Robert Israel. "Bowel Obstruction and Perforation with an Intraperitoneal Loop Intrauterine Contraceptive Device." *American Journal of Obstetrics and Gynecology* 129 (1977): 461–62.

D'Arcy, Patrick Francis, and J. P. Griffin. *Iatrogenic Disease*. London: Oxford University Press, 1972.

Dashow, Edward E., and Alfred S. Lorens. "Resistant Gonococcal Infection from an Intrauterine Contraceptive Device." *American Journal of Obstetrics and Gynecology* 129 (1977): 230.

Davis, Hugh J. "Intrauterine Contraceptive Devices: Present Status and Future Prospects." *American Journal of Obstetrics and Gynecology* 114 (1972): 134–51.

———. *Intrauterine Devices for Contraception: The IUD*. Baltimore: Williams and Wilkins, 1971.

———. "The Shield Intrauterine Device: A Superior Modern Contraceptive." *American Journal of Obstetrics and Gynecology* 106 (1970): 455–62.

Davis, Hugh J., and John Lesinski. "Mechanisms of Action of Intrauterine Contraceptives in Women." *Obstetrics and Gynecology* 36 (1970): 350–58.

Debancens, Alfredo, Rodrigo Prado, Raul Larraguibel, and Juan Ranartu. "Intrapithelial Cervical Neoplasia in Women Using Intrauterine Devices and Long-Acting Injectable Progestins and Contraceptives." *American Journal of Obstetrics and Gynecology* 119 (1974): 1052–56.

Delaney, D., B. Fonget, L. Myers, and P. Thorn. "Androgenisation of Female Partners of Men on Medroxyprogesterone Acetate Percutaneous Testosterone Contraception." *The Lancet*, February 4, 1984, 276.

Demarest, Robert J., and John J. Sciarra. *Conception, Birth and Contraception: A Visual Presentation*. New York: McGraw-Hill, 1976.

Denes, Magda. *In Necessity and Sorrow: Life and Death in an Abortion Hospital*. New York: Penguin, 1977.

"Development of Six New Contraceptives among 1989 Goals of WHO Programme." *Family Planning Perspectives* 15/5 (1983): 226–27.

De Young, P., J. Martyn, H. Wass, L. Hartl, E. Crichton, and C. Reynolds. "Toxic Shock Syndrome Associated with a Contraceptive Diaphragm." *Canadian Medical Association Journal* 127 (1982): 611–12.

Dhall, Kamla, G. I. Dhall, and Brij Bala Gupta. "Uterine Perforation with the Lippes Loop: Detection by Hysterography." *Obstetrics and Gynecology* 34 (1969): 266–70.

Diaz, S., H. B. Croxatto, and M. Panez. "Clinical Chemistry in Women Treated with Six Levonorgestral Covered Rods or with a Copper IUD." *Contraception* 31 (1985): 321–31.

Dick-Read, Grantly. *Childbirth without Fear*. 4th ed. New York: Harper and Row, 1978 (originally published 1949).

Diczfalucy, Egon. "New Developments in Oral Injectable and Implantable Contraceptives, Vaginal Rings and Intrauterine Devices: A Review." *Contraception* 33 (1986): 7–23.

Diddle, A. W., William H. Gardner, and Perry J. Williamson. "Oral Contraceptive Medications and Headache." *American Journal of Obstetrics and Gynecology* 105 (1969): 507–11.

Dienes, C. Thomas. *Law, Politics and Birth Control*. Urbana: University of Illinois Press, 1972.

Di Paola, G., F. Puchulu, M. Robin, R. Nicholson, and M. Marti. "Oral Contraceptives and Carbohydrate Metabolism." *American Journal of Obstetrics and Gynecology* 101 (1968): 106–16.

Di Saia, Philip J., and C. Paul Morrow. "Unusual Side Effect of Megistrol Acetate." *American Journal of Obstetrics and Gynecology* 129 (1977): 460–61.

Djerassi, Carl. *The Politics of Contraception*. New York: W.W. Norton, 1979.

Donovan, Patricia. "Airing Contraceptive Commercials." *Family Planning Perspectives* 14/6 (1982): 321–23.

———. "Wrongful Birth and Wrongful Conception: The Legal and Moral Issues." *Family Planning Perspectives* 16/2 (1984): 64–69.

"Doubts about the Pill." *Newsweek*, May 19, 1969, 118.

Dowie, Mark. "The Corporate Crime of the Century." *Mother Jones*, November 1979.

Draper, Bernard, and Eugene F. White. "Puerperal Insertion of the Dalkon Shield: A Private Patient Experience." *American Journal of Obstetrics and Gynecology* 115 (1973): 278–79.

Dreishpoon, Irving H. "Complications of Pregnancy with an Intrauterine Contraceptive Device in Situ." *American Journal of Obstetrics and Gynecology* 121 (1975): 412–13.

Duffy, Benedict J., Jr., and Sister M. Jean Wallace. *Biological and Medical Aspects of Contraception*. London: University of Notre Dame Press, 1969.

Dworkin, Andrea. *Intercourse*. New York: Free Press, 1987.

"Ectopic Pregnancy and IUD's." *FDA Consumer*, March 1979, 2.

Edelman, David A. "Dalkon Shield Tails." *Fertility and Sterility* 41 (1984): 159–61.

———. "Vaginal Contraception: An Overview." *International Journal of Gynecology and Obstetrics* 22 (1984): 11–17.

Edelman, David A., Louis Keith, and Gary S. Berger. "Intrauterine Devices and Pelvic Inflammatory Disease." *Journal of the American Medical Association* 251 (1984): 1278–79.

Ehrenreich, Barbara. *The Hearts of Men*. New York: Anchor, 1984.

Ehrenreich, Barbara, Mark Dowie, and Stephen Minkin. "The Charge: Gynocide; the Accused: The U.S. Government." *Mother Jones*, November 1979.

Ehrenreich, Barbara, and Dierdre English. *Complaints and Disorders: The Sexual Politics of Sickness*. Old Westbury, N.Y.: Feminist Press, 1973.

———. *For Her Own Good: 150 Years of the Experts' Advice to Women*. Garden City, N.Y.: Anchor, 1979.

———. *Witches, Midwives and Nurses: A History of Women Healers*. Old Westbury, N.Y.: Feminist, Press, 1973.

Eisinger, Steven H. "Second-Trimester Spontaneous Abortion, the IUD, and Infection." *American Journal of Obstetrics and Gynecology* 124 (1976): 393–97.

Elias, Julian. "Intra-Uterine Contraceptive Devices." *The Practitioner* 229 (1985): 431–36.

El-Mahgoub, S. "D-Norgestral Slow-Releasing T Device as an Intrauterine Contraceptive." *American Journal of Obstetrics and Gynecology* 123 (1975): 133–38.

Elstein, Max. "The Present Status of Contraception." *The Practitioner* 208 (1972): 485–92.

Engineer, Amy D., Jata S. Misra, and Prabha Tandon. "Comparative Cytologic Evaluation of Device Smears in Women Using CuT 200 Devices and Lippes Loop." *Indian Journal of Medical Research* 79 (1984): 766–71.

———. "Long-Term Cytologic Studies of Copper-IUD Users." *Acta Cytologica* 25 (1981): 550–56.

Esposito, John M. "Perforation of the Uterus Secondary to Insertion of IUCD." *Obstetrics and Gynecology* 28 (1966): 799–805.

Esposito, John M., Donald M. Zaron, and George S. Zaron. "A Dalkon Shield Imbedded in a Myoma: Case Report of an Unusual Displacement of an Intrauterine Device." *American Journal of Obstetrics and Gynecology* 117 (1973): 578–81.

"Estrogens: Enough to Move FDA." *Science News* 97 (1970): 430–31.

Evans, Barbara. *Freedom to Choose: The Life and Work of Dr. Helena Wright, Pioneer of Contraception.* London: Bradley House, 1984.

Faden, Alan, Jean-Paul Spire, and Ruth Faden. "Fits, Faints, and the IUD." *Annals of Neurology* 1 (1977): 305–06.

Faundes, Anibal, Sheldon J. Segal, Christopher A. Adejuwon, Vivian Brache, Patricia Leon, and Francisco Alvarez-Sanchez. "The Menstrual Cycle in Women Using an Intrauterine Device." *Fertility and Sterility* 34 (1980): 427–30.

"FDA Approves Injectable Contraceptive for Limited Use in Women." *FDA Consumer,* December 1973–January 1974, 29.

"FDA Okays Limited Use of Injectable Contraceptive." *Journal of the American Medical Association* 226 (1973): 734.

"FDA Unit Urges Ban on A. H. Robins' IUD Continue until Study." *Wall Street Journal,* August 26, 1974, 14.

Federation of Feminist Women's Health Centers. *A New View of a Woman's Body.* New York: Simon and Schuster, 1981.

Field, Marilyn Jane. *The Comparative Politics of Birth Control: Determinants of Policy Variation and Change in the Developed Nations.* New York: Praeger, 1983.

"Final Warning?" *Newsweek,* June 22, 1970, 76.

"The First Complete Guide to Modern Birth Control." *Ladies' Home Journal,* July 1967, 43–45.

Fisher, Sue. *In the Patient's Best Interest: Women and the Politics of Medical Decisions.* New Brunswick: Rutgers University Press, 1988.

Forrest, Jacqueline Darroch. "The End of IUD Marketing in the United States: What Does It Mean for American Women?" *Family Planning Perspectives* 18/2 (1986): 52–57.

Fortier, Lise, Yves Lefebvre, Michael LaRose, and Robert Lanctat. "Canadian Experience with a Copper-Covered Intrauterine Contraceptive Device." *American Journal of Obstetrics and Gynecology* 115 (1973): 291–97.

Frankfort, Ellen. *Vaginal Politics.* New York: Quadrangle, 1972.

Fraser, Ian S. "A Survey of Different Approaches to Management of Menstrual Disturbances in Women Using Injectable Contraceptives." *Contraception* 28 (1983): 385–97.

Fraser, Ian S., and Edith Weisberg. "Fertility Following Discontinuation of Different Methods of Fertility Control." *Contraception* 26 (1982): 389–403.

Fraser, Ian S., and Robert P. S. Jansen. "Why Do Inadvertent Pregnancies Occur in Oral Contraceptive Users? Effectiveness of Oral Contraceptive Regimens and Interfering Factors." *Contraception* 27 (1983): 531–51.

Freid, John F. *Vasectomy: The Truth and Consequences of the Newest Form of Birth Control—Male Sterilization.* New York: Saturday Review Press, 1972.

Friedan, Betty. *The Second Stage.* New York: Summit, 1981.

Gallegos, Alfredo J. "The Zoapatle I—A Traditional Remedy from Mexico Emerges to Modern Times." *Contraception* 27 (1983): 211–21.

Garcia, Celso-Ramon. "What's Sure besides the Pill?" *Redbook,* January, 1970, 341.

Gibor, Yair, and Constance Mitchell. "Selected Events Following Insertion of the Progestasert® System." *Contraception* 21 (1980): 491–503.

Gibson, Mark, Dieter Gump, Taka Ashikaga, and Bruce Hall. "Patterns of Adnexal Inflammatory Damage: Chlamydia, the Intrauterine Device, and History of Pelvic Inflammatory Disease." *Fertility and Sterility* 41 (1984): 47–51.

Gillespie, Larrian. "The Diaphragm: An Accomplice in Recurrent Urinary Tract Infections." *Urology* 24 (1984): 25–30.

Glaser, Barney G., and Anselm L. Strauss. *The Discovery of Grounded Theory: Strategies for Qualitative Research.* Chicago: Aldine, 1967.

Glass, Robert H., and Nathan Kase. *Woman's Choice: A Guide to Contraception, Fertility, Abortion and Menopause.* New York: Basic Books, 1970.

Goh, T. H., and M. Harihan. "Effect of Laparoscopic Sterilization and Insertion of Multiload Cu250 and Progestasert IUDs on Serum Ferritin Levels." *Contraception* 28 (1983): 329–34.

Gold, Rachel Benson. "Depo-Provera: The Jury Still Out." *International Family Planning Perspectives* 9 (1983): 15–18.

Golde, Steven H., Robert Israel, and William J. Ledger. "Unilateral Tubovarian Abscess: A Distinct Entity." *American Journal of Obstetrics and Gynecology* 127 (1977): 807–10.

Golden, A. S. "Umbilical Cord–Placental Separation: A Complication of IUD Failure." *Journal of Reproductive Medicine* 11 (1973): 79–80.

Goldenthal, Edwin I. "Contraceptives, Estrogens and Progestogens: A New FDA Policy on Animal Studies." *FDA Papers,* November 1969, 15.

Golditch, Ira M., and James E. Huston. "Serious Pelvic Infections Associated with Intrauterine Contraceptive Device." *International Journal of Fertility* 18 (1973): 156–60.

Goldman, J. A., D. Peleg, D. Feldberg, D. Dicker, and N. Samuel. "Case Report: IUD Appendicitis." *European Journal of Obstetrics, Gynecology, and Reproductive Biology* 15 (1983): 181–83.

Goldstein, Leopold Z. "Control of Conception: The Use Effectiveness of a New Cream-Jel." *Obstetrics and Gynecology* 10 (1957): 133–39.

Goldstein, Marc, and Nicki Fieldberg. *The Vasectomy Book: A Guide to Decision Making.* Los Angeles: J. P. Tarcher, 1982.

Goldzieher, Joseph W. "New Report on Oral Contraceptives of the Advisory Committee to the Food and Drug Administration: A Comment on the New Report." *American Journal of Obstetrics and Gynecology* 107 (1970): 1106–07.

Goldzieher, Joseph W., and Lazewell S. Dozier. "Oral Contraceptives and Thromboembolism: A Reassessment." *American Journal of Obstetrics and Gynecology* 123 (1975): 878–914.

Goldzieher, Joseph W., Lonis E. Moses, Eugene Averkin, Cora Schul, and Ben Z. Faber. "Nervousness and Depression Attributed to Oral Contraceptives: A Double-Blind, Placebo-Controlled Study." *American Journal of Obstetrics and Gynecology* 111 (1971): 1013–20.

Goldzieher, Joseph W., and Harry W. Rudel. "How the Oral Contraceptives Came to Be Developed." *Journal of the American Medical Association* 230 (1974): 421–25.

Gordon, Arthur. "Birth Control Success Story No. 1." *Reader's Digest,* January 1970, 80–84. (Condensed from *Today's Health*)

Gordon, Jeoffrey. "Oral Contraceptives: Risks and Benefits." *New England Journal of Medicine* 289 (1973): 809.

Gordon, Linda. "The Struggle for Reproductive Freedom: Three Stages of Feminism."

In *Capitalist Patriarchy and the Case for Socialist Feminism*, ed. Zillah Eisenstein, 107–32. New York: Monthly Review Press, 1979.

———. *Woman's Body, Woman's Right*. New York: Penguin, 1977.

Gordon, Philippa H., and Laurie J. De Marco. "Reproductive Health Services for Men: Is There a Need?" *Family Planning Perspectives* 16/1 (1984): 44–49.

"Gossypol." *Journal of the American Medical Association* 252 (1984): 1102–03.

"Gossypol Prospects." *The Lancet,* May 19, 1984, 1108–09.

Gould, Stephen J. *The Mismeasure of Man*. New York: W.W. Norton, 1981.

Graff, Giora, Moshe Lancet, and Bernard Czernobilsky. "Ovarian Pregnancy with Intrauterine Devices in Situ." *Obstetrics and Gynecology* 40 (1972): 535–38.

Graham, Sian, and Barbara Simcock. "A Review of the Use of Intrauterine Devices in Nulliparous Women." *Contraception* 26 (1982): 323–46.

Grant, Ellen. *The Bitter Pill: How Safe Is the "Perfect Contraceptive"?* London: Elm Tree, 1985.

Gray, Cyrus L., and Eugene H. Ruffolo. "Ovarian Pregnancy Associated with Intra-uterine Contraceptive Devices." *American Journal of Obstetrics and Gynecology* 132 (1978): 134–39.

Green, Shirley. *The Curious History of Contraception*. New York: St. Martin's, 1971.

Greenfield, Natalie S. *"First Do No Harm": A Dying Woman's Battle against the Physicians and Drug Companies Who Misled Her about the Hazards of the Pill*. New York: Sun River, 1976.

Greer, Germaine. *Sex and Destiny: The Politics of Human Fertility*. New York: Harper and Row, 1984.

Grele, Ron. *Envelopes of Sound: The Art of Oral History*. 2d ed. Chicago: Precedent, 1985.

Grobowski, Henry G., and John M. Vernon. *The Regulation of Pharmaceuticals: Balancing the Benefits and Risks*. Washington: American Enterprise Institute for Public Policy Research, 1983.

Gruer, Laurence. "Risks of Intrauterine Contraceptive Devices." *British Medical Journal* 288 (1984): 1919.

Gruer, Laurence D., K. E. Collingsham, and C. W. Edwards. "Pneuomococcal Peritonitis Associated with an IUD." *The Lancet,* September 17, 1983, 677.

Guderian, A. Maynard, and Gerald E. Trobough. "Residues of Pelvic Inflammatory Disease in Intrauterine Device Users: A Result of the Intrauterine Device or Chlamydia Trachomatis Infection?" *American Journal of Obstetrics and Gynecology* 154 (1986): 497–503.

Guha-Ray, Dilip K. "Translocation of the Intrauterine Contraceptive Device. Study of Thirty-One Cases." *Fertility and Sterility* 28 (1977): 943–46.

Guidoin, Robert, James M. Courtney, Roger Brault, Dominique Domurado, and Geoffrey H. Haggis. "Intra-Uterine Devices: A SEM Study on the Dalkon Shield." *Biomaterials, Medical Devices and Artificial Organs: An International Journal* 4 (1976): 81–117.

Gusdon, John P. "An Immunologic Method of Pregnancy Destruction and Contraception." *American Journal of Obstetrics and Gynecology* 112 (1972): 472–75.

Guttmacher, Alan F. *Birth Control and Love: The Complete Guide to Contraception and Fertility*. 2d rev. ed. London: Macmillan, 1969.

———. "How to Succeed at Family Planning: A World-Famous Authority Evaluates Current Birth Control Methods." *Parents Magazine,* January 1969.

Guttmacher, Alan F., Winfield Best, and Frederic C. Jaffe. *Planning Your Family: The Complete Guide to Contraception and Fertility.* New York: Macmillan, 1964.

"Gynex Oral Contraceptives Recalled." *FDA Consumer,* June 1987, 6.

Hackett, Robert E., and Keith Waterhance. "Vasectomy—Reviewed." *American Journal of Obstetrics and Gynecology* 116 (1973): 438–55.

Haire, Doris. *How the FDA Determines the "Safety" of Drugs—Just How Safe Is "Safe"? A Report Released to the Congress of the United States.* Washington: National Women's Health Network, 1984.

Hall, Herbert H., Alexander Sedlis, Irvin Chabon, and Martin L. Stone. "Effect of Intrauterine Stainless Steel Ring on Endometrial Structure and Function." *American Journal of Obstetrics and Gynecology* 93 (1965): 1031–41.

Hall, Robert E. "A Comparative Evaluation of Intrauterine Contraceptive Devices." *American Journal of Obstetrics and Gynecology* 94 (1966): 65–77.

———. "A Reappraisal of Intrauterine Contraceptive Devices: Prompted by the Delayed Discovery of Uterine Perforations." *American Journal of Obstetrics and Gynecology* 99 (1967): 808–13.

———. "Therapeutic Abortion, Sterilization and Contraception." *American Journal of Obstetrics and Gynecology* 91 (1965): 518–32.

Hallatt, Jack G. "Ectopic Pregnancy Associated with the Intrauterine Device: A Study of Seventy Cases." *American Journal of Obstetrics and Gynecology* 125 (1976): 755–58.

Hardin, Garrett. *Birth Control.* New York: Pegasus, 1970.

Harding, Sandra. *Feminism and Methodology.* Indianapolis: Indiana University Press, 1987.

Harris, W. H. "Complications of the IUD." *Canadian Medical Journal* 119 (1973): 677.

Harrison, Beverly Wildung. *Our Right to Choose: Toward a New Ethic of Abortion.* Boston: Beacon, 1983.

Harrison, Michelle. *A Woman in Residence.* New York: Penguin, 1982.

Hartmann, Betsy. *Reproductive Rights and Wrongs: The Global Politics of Population Control and Contraceptive Choice.* New York: Harper and Row, 1987.

Hartmann, Heidi. "Changes in Women's Economic and Family Roles in Post–World War II United States." In *Women, Households and the Economy,* ed. Lourdes Beneira and Catherine A. Stimpson, 33–64. New Brunswick: Rutgers University Press. 1987.

"Having a Baby inside Me Is the Only Time I'm Really Alive." In *The Black Woman in White America,* ed. Gerda Lerner, 313. New York: Vintage, 1973.

Hawkins, D. F. "Intrauterine Contraception." *The Practitioner* 205 (1970): 20.

Heinonen, P. K., M. Merikari, and J. Paavonen. "Uterine Perforation by Copper Intrauterine Device." *European Journal of Obstetrics, Gynecology, and Reproductive Medicine* 17 (1984): 260.

Helmrich, Susan P., Lynn Rosenberg, David W. Kaufman, Brian Strom, and Samuel Shapiro. "Venous Thromboembolism in Relation to Oral Contraceptive Use." *Obstetrics and Gynecology* 69 (1987): 91–95.

Henderson, Simon R. "Pelvic Actinomycosis Associated with an Intrauterine Device." *Obstetrics and Gynecology* 41 (1973): 726–32.

Herbert, Timothy J., and P. P. Mortimer. "Recurrent Pneumococcal Peritonitis Associated with an Intra-Uterine Contraceptive Device." *British Journal of Surgery* 61 (1974): 901–02.

Hester, Lawrence L., Jr., W. W. Kellett III, Samuel S. Spicer, H. Oliver Williamson, and H. R. Pratt-Thomas. "Effects of a Sequential Oral Contraceptive on Endometrial Enzyme and Carbohydrate Histochemistry." *American Journal of Obstetrics and Gynecology* 102 (1968): 771–83.

Himes, Norman. *Medical History of Contraception.* New York: Gamut, 1936.

Hite, Shere. *The Hite Report: A Nationwide Study of Female Sexuality.* Rev. ed. New York: Dell, 1981.

———. *The Hite Report on Male Sexuality: How Men Feel about Love, Sex, and Relationships.* New York: Ballantine, 1982.

———. *Women and Love: A Cultural Revolution in Progress.* New York: Alfred A. Knopf, 1987.

Hobel, Calvin J., and Daniel R. Mishell, Jr. "Pulmonary Embolism and Oral Steroidal Contraceptives." *American Journal of Obstetrics and Gynecology* 101 (1968): 994–96.

Hochner-Celnikier, Drorith, Ariel Milwidsky, Moshe Menashe, Ilena Ariel, and Zvi Palti. "Pelvic Abscess Associated with a Lippes Loop: An Unusual Case." *Journal of Reproductive Medicine* 28 (1983): 542–45.

Holmes, Helen B., Betty B. Hoskins, and Michael Gross, eds. *Birth Control and Controlling Birth: Woman-Centered Perspectives.* Clifton, N.J.: Humana, 1980.

"Hormonal Contraceptives: Long-Acting Methods." *Population Reports,* ser. K, no. 3 (vol. 15/1). Baltimore: Johns Hopkins University, Population Information Program, 1987.

Illich, Iman D. *Medical Nemesis: The Expropriation of Health.* New York: Pantheon, 1976.

"Informing Women about 'The Pill.'" *FDA Consumer,* February 1977, 20–21.

International Planned Parenthood Federation. *Family Planning Handbook for Doctors.* London: IPPF, 1974.

"Intrauterine Contraceptive Devices." *Drug and Therapeutics Bulletin,* August 17, 1983, 65–68.

"Intrauterine Devices: Precautions during Use." *California Medicine, the Western Journal of Medicine* 19/4 (1973): 85–86.

Isaacs, John H., and John S. O'Connor. "Treatment of Tubal Pregnancy." *Obstetrics and Gynecology* 23 (1964): 187–91.

Ishihama, Atsumi, and Teruo Kasabu. "Cytological Studies after Insertion of Intrauterine Contraceptive Devices." *American Journal of Obstetrics and Gynecology* 91 (1965): 576–78.

Ismail, A.A.A., M. Y. Anwar, S. M. Youssef, and M. Toppozada. "Ovulation Detection Following Removal of Levonorgestrel Subdermal Contraceptive Implants." *Contraception* 35 (1987): 207–14.

"IUD's—A New Look." *Population Reports,* ser. B, no. 5 (vol. 16/1). Baltimore: Johns Hopkins University, Population Information Program, 1988.

Jewett, John Figgis. "Chorio-Amnionitis Complicated by an Intrauterine Device." *New England Journal of Medicine* 289 (1973): 1251–52.

Johnson, Jeannette H. "Vasectomy: An International Appraisal." *Family Planning Perspectives* 15/1 (1983): 45–48.

Johnson, William L., Theodore W. Ek, and Larry L. Brewer. "Mobility of the Human Uterus before and after Insertion of an Intrauterine Device." *Obstetrics and Gynecology* 28 (1966): 526–27.

Jones, Georgeanna Seegar. "Women—The Impact of Advances in Fertility Control on Their Future: A Presidential Address." *Fertility and Sterility* 22 (1971): 347–50.

Jones, Mary C., Bruce O. Buschmann, Edmund A. Dowling, and Helen M. Pollock. "The Prevalence of Actinomycetis-like Organisms Found in Cervicovaginal Smears of 300 IUD Wearers." *Acta Cytologica* 23 (1979): 282–86.

Jones, R. W., A. Parker, and Max Elstein. "Clinical Experience with the Dalkon Shield Intrauterine Device." *British Medical Journal,* July 21, 1973, 143–45.

Josey, William E., Willis Hoch, Elliott C. Moon, and John D. Thompson. "An Analysis of 21 Septic Abortion Deaths with Special Reference to the Schwartzman Phenomenon." *Obstetrics and Gynecology* 28 (1966): 335–41.

Kafka, Denise, and Rachel Benson Gold. "Food and Drug Administration Approves Vaginal Sponge." *Family Planning Perspectives* 15/3 (1983): 146–47.

Kahn, Henry S., and Carl W. Tyler, Jr. "An Association between the Dalkon Shield and Complicated Pregnancies among Women Hospitalized for Intrauterine Contraceptive Device–Related Disorders." *American Journal of Obstetrics and Gynecology* 125 (1976): 83–86.

"Kaiser Study Links 'Pill' and Risk of Hypertension." *Journal of the American Medical Association* 228 (1974): 17–18.

Kane, Francis J., Jr. "Psychiatric Reactions to Oral Contraceptives." *American Journal of Obstetrics and Gynecology* 102 (1968): 1059–62.

Kapur, M. M., S. Mokkapati, A. Faroq, R. K. Ahsan, and K. R. Laumas. "Copper Intravas Device (IVD) and Male Contraception." *Contraception* 29 (1984): 45–54.

Kar, Amiya B., Amy D. Engineer, P. R. Dasgupta, and A. K. Srivastava. "Effect of an Intrauterine Contraceptive Device on Urea Content of Uterine Fluid." *American Journal of Obstetrics and Gynecology* 104 (1969): 607–08.

Kar, Amiya B., Amy D. Engineer, Rashmi Goel, V. P. Kamboj, P. R. Dasgupta, and S. R. Chowdhury. "Effect of an Intrauterine Contraceptive Device on Biochemical Composition of Uterine Fluid." *American Journal of Obstetrics and Gynecology* 101 (1968): 966–70.

Kar, Amiya B., B. S. Selty, and V. P. Kamboj. "Postcoital Contraception by Topical Application of Some Steroidal and Nonsteroidal Agents." *American Journal of Obstetrics and Gynecology* 102 (1968): 306–07.

Karrer, Max C., and Edward R. Smith. "Two Thousand Woman-Years' Experience with a Sequential Contraceptive: A More Effective Method of Taking a Sequential Contraceptive." *American Journal of Obstetrics and Gynecology* 102 (1968): 1029–34.

Kaufman, David W., Jane Watson, Lynn Rosenberg, Susan P. Helmrich, Donald R. Miller, Olli S. Miettinen, Paul D. Stolley, and Samuel Shapiro. "The Effect of Different Types of Intrauterine Devices on the Risk of Pelvic Inflammatory Disease." *Journal of the American Medical Association* 250 (1983): 759–62.

Kelaghan, Joseph, George L. Rubin, Howard W. Ory, and Peter Layde. "Barrier Method Contraceptives and Pelvic Inflammatory Disease." *Journal of the American Medical Association* 248 (1982): 184–87.

Kelly, John, and Janice Aaron. "Pelvic Actinomycosis and Usage of Intrauterine Contraceptive Devices." *Yale Journal of Biology and Medicine* 55 (1982): 453–61.

Kendall, W. "The IUD and PID." *Canadian Medical Association Journal* 115 (1976): 20.

Kerber, Linda K. "Separate Spheres, Female Worlds, Woman's Place: The Rhetoric of Women's History." *Journal of American History* 75 (1988): 9–39.

Kim, Doo-Sung, Youn-Yeung Hwang, Kil-Chun Kang, and Moon-Il Park. "Migration of the Lippes Loop into the Fallopian Tube." *Obstetrics and Gynecology* 60 (1982): 393–94.

Kirk, R. Mark. "Ureteral Obstruction Complicating the IUD." *Journal of the American Medical Association* 215 (1971): 1156.

Kisnisci, Husnu, and Cheryle B. Champion. "A Study of Delta Intrauterine Devices in Ankara, Turkey." *International Journal of Obstetrics and Gynecology* 23 (1985): 51–54.

Kistner, Robert W. *The Pill.* New York: Delacorte, 1969.

———. "Questions Women Ask Most about 'the Pill.'" *Good Housekeeping,* February 1969, 78–79.

———. *Uses of Progestin in Obstetrics and Gynecology.* Chicago: Year Book Medical Publishers, 1969.

———. "What 'the Pill' Does to Husbands." *Ladies' Home Journal,* January 1969, 66.

Kitzinger, Sheila. *Woman's Experience of Sex: The Facts and Feelings of Female Sexuality at Every Stage of Life.* New York: Penguin, 1985.

Kivijarvi, A., H. Jarvinen, and M. Gronroos. "Microbiology of Vaginitis Associated with the Intrauterine Contraceptive Device." *British Journal of Obstetrics and Gynecology* 91 (1984): 917–23.

Klaus, Hanna. "Natural Family Planning." *FDA Consumer,* September 1982, 2.

Klitsch, Michael. "Hormonal Implants: The Next Wave of Contraceptives." *Family Planning Perspectives* 15/5 (1983): 239–43.

Knoch, M. H. "Intrauterine Contraceptive Devices." *American Journal of Obstetrics and Gynecology* 116 (1973): 589–90.

———. "A New Intrauterine Contraceptive Device." *American Journal of Obstetrics and Gynecology* 99 (1967): 428–30.

Kohl, Schuyler. "Is Pregnancy the Time to Think about Spacing Children?" *Redbook,* November 1967, 29–32.

Korenbrat, Carol. "Value Conflicts in Biomedical Research into Future Contraceptives." In *Birth Control and Controlling Birth: Woman-Centered Perspectives,* ed. Helen B. Holmes, Betty B. Hoskins, and Michael Gross, 47–54. Clifton, N.J.: Humana, 1980.

Kothari, M. L., and D. S. Pardanani. "Temporary Sterilization of the Male (Human Subject) by an Intravasal Contraceptive Device (IVCD)." *Journal of Reproduction and Fertility* 17 (1971): 292.

Lader, Laurence. "Why Birth Control Fails." *McCall's,* October 1969, 75.

Lake, Alice. "The Pill: What We Really Know after 15 Years of Use." *McCall's,* January 1975, 76–77.

Lambert, Edward C. *Modern Medical Mistakes.* Bloomington: Indiana University Press, 1978.

Lane, Mary E., Emilia Dacalos, Aquiles J. Sobrero, and William B. Ober. "Squamous Metaplasia of the Endometrium in Women with an Intrauterine Contraceptive Device: Follow-Up Study." *American Journal of Obstetrics and Gynecology* 119 (1974): 693–97.

Lauersen, Niels H., Lars L. Cederqvist, Susan Donovan, and Fritz Fuchs. "Comparison of Three Intrauterine Contraceptive Devices: The Antigon-F, the Ypsilon-Y, and the Copper T200." *Fertility and Sterility* 26 (1975): 639–48.

Lautt, M. E. "Complication of I.U.D." *New England Journal of Medicine* 283 (1970): 1350.

Layde, Peter M. "Pelvic Inflammatory Disease and the Dalkon Shield." *Journal of the American Medical Association* 250 (1983): 796–97.

Layde, Peter M., Howard W. Ory, and James J. Schlesselman. "The Risk of Myocardial Infarction in Former Users of Oral Contraceptives." *Family Planning Perspectives* 14/2 (1982): 78–80.

Leader, Abel J. "The Houston Story: A Vasectomy Service in a Family Planning Clinic." *Family Planning Perspectives* 3/3 (1971): 46–49.

Ledger, William J., and Frank J. Schrader. "Death from Septicemia Following Insertion of an Intrauterine Device: Report of a Case." *Obstetrics and Gynecology* 31 (1968): 845–48.

Ledger, William J., and J. Robert Willson. "Intrauterine Contraceptive Devices: The Recognition and Management of Uterine Perforations." *Obstetrics and Gynecology* 28 (1966): 806–11.

Lee, C. H., L. P. Chow, F. Y. Cheng, and P. Y. Wei. "Histologic Study of the Endometrium of Intrauterine Contraceptive Device Users." *American Journal of Obstetrics and Gynecology* 98 (1967): 808–10.

Lee, Nancy C., George L. Rubin, Howard W. Ory, and Ronald L. Burkman. "Type of Intrauterine Device and the Risk of Pelvic Inflammatory Disease." *Obstetrics and Gynecology* 62 (1983): 1–6.

Lee, Raymond A. "Contraceptive and Endometrial Effects of Medroxyprogesterone Acetate." *American Journal of Obstetrics and Gynecology* 104 (1969): 130–33.

Leiman, Gladwyn. "Depomedroxyprogesterone Acetate as a Contraceptive Agent: Its Effect on Weight and Blood Pressure." *American Journal of Obstetrics and Gynecology* 114 (1972): 97–101.

Leventhal, John M., Lenard R. Simion, and Sander S. Shapiro. "Laparoscopic Removal of Intrauterine Contraceptive Devices Following Uterine Perforation." *American Journal of Obstetrics and Gynecology* 111 (1971): 102–05.

Levin, S., E. Caspi, and H. Hirsch. "Ovarian Pregnancy and Intrauterine Devices." *American Journal of Obstetrics and Gynecology* 113 (1972): 843–44.

Levinson, Carl, and David C. Richardson. "The Dalkon Shield Story." *Advances in Planned Parenthood* 11/2 (1976): 53–63.

Lin, T. J., Y. Tanaka, Ramon Aznar, S. C. Lin, Y. Yamasaki, S. Hori, H. K. Brar, Kenneth T. Kirton, and B. Little. "Contraceptive Effect of Intrauterine Application of Lugol's Solution." *American Journal of Obstetrics and Gynecology* 116 (1973): 167–74.

Lindsay, Colton M., ed. *The Pharmaceutical Industry: Economics, Performance, and Government Regulation.* New York: John Wiley and Sons, 1978.

Liner, Robert. "Ectopic Pregnancy." *Obstetrics and Gynecology* 64 (1984): 297–300.

Lippes, Jack. "Contraception with Intrauterine Plastic Loops." *American Journal of Obstetrics and Gynecology* 93 (1965): 1024–30.

"Long-Acting Progestins—Promise and Prospects." *Population Reports*, ser. K, no. 2 (vol.

11/2). Baltimore: Johns Hopkins University, Population Information Program, 1983.

Low, Setha M., and Bruce C. Newman. "Indigenous Fertility Regulating Methods in Costa Rica." In *Women's Medicine,* ed. Lucile F. Newman, 147–60. New Brunswick: Rutgers University Press, 1985.

Luker, Kristin. *Abortion and the Politics of Motherhood.* Berkeley: University of California Press, 1984.

———. *Taking Chances: Abortion and the Decision Not to Contracept.* Berkeley: University of California Press, 1975.

Luukkainen, Tapani, Hanna Allonen, Maija Haukkamaa, Pertti Lahteenmaki, Carl Gustaf Nilsson, and Juhani Toivoner. "Five Years' Experience with Levonorgestrel-Releasing IUDs." *Contraception* 33 (1986): 139–49.

McCammon, Robert E. "The Birnberg Bow as an Intrauterine Contraceptive Device." *Obstetrics and Gynecology* 29 (1967): 67–69.

MacCorquadale, Patricia L. "Gender Roles and Premarital Contraception." *Journal of Marriage and the Family* (February 1984): 57–63.

McDonnell, Kathleen. *Adverse Effects: Women and the Pharmaceutical Industry.* Toronto: Women's Educational Press, 1986.

McElin, Thomas W. "Severe Peritonitis and the IUD." *American Journal of Obstetrics and Gynecology* 113 (1972): 570.

McGill, Michael E. *The McGill Report on Male Intimacy.* New York: Harper and Row, 1986.

MacIntyre, Susan L., and James E. Higgins. "Parity and Use-Effectiveness with the Contraceptive Sponge." *American Journal of Obstetrics and Gynecology* 155 (1986): 798–801.

McQuarrie, Howard G., Charles D. Scott, Homer D. Ellsworth, John W. Harris, and Rodney A. Stone. "Cytogenic Studies in Women Using Oral Contraceptives and Their Progeny." *American Journal of Obstetrics and Gynecology* 108 (1970): 659–65.

"Majzlin Spring IUDs Seized in New York." *FDA Consumer,* September 1973, 26.

Makblonf, Aly Marei, and Ahmed Fawzy Abdel-Salam. "Kymographic Studies of the Fallopian Tubes after Insertion of Intrauterine Contraceptive Devices Using the Lippes Loop and the Nylon Ring." *American Journal of Obstetrics and Gynecology* 106 (1970): 759–64.

Malony, W. R., and Joseph P. Meranti. "Ectopic Pregnancy and the Intrauterine Device." *Journal of the American College Health Association* 21 (1972): 167–68.

Margolis, Alan J. "A Fluid-Filled Intrauterine Device: Initial Clinical Trials." *American Journal of Obstetrics and Gynecology* 122 (1975): 470–75.

Margulies, Lazar C. "Intrauterine Contraception: A New Approach." *Obstetrics and Gynecology* 24 (1964): 515–20.

Marquez-Monter, Hector, C. Francisco Funes, Ramon Aznar, Juan Giner-Velazquez, and Jorge Martinez-Mavtauton. "In Vitro Autoradiographic Study of the Endometrium from Women Treated with Low-Dose Chlormadinone Acetate for Contraception." *American Journal of Obstetrics and Gynecology* 102 (1968): 896–900.

Marshall, Byrne R., James K. Hepler, and Masaharu S. Jinguji. "Fatal Streptococcus Pyogenes Septicemia Associated with an Intrauterine Device." *Obstetrics and Gynecology* 41 (1973): 83–87.

Massouras, H. G. "Intrauterine Adhesions: A Syndrome of the Past with the Use of the Massouras Duck's Foot No. 2 Intrauterine Contraceptive Device." *American Journal of Obstetrics and Gynecology* 116 (1973): 576–79.

"Maternal Deaths and the IUD." *The Lancet,* December 4, 1976, 1234–35.

Mead, Philip B., Jackson B. Beecham, and John Van S. Maeck. "Incidence of Infections Associated with the Intrauterine Contraceptive Device in an Isolated Community." *American Journal of Obstetrics and Gynecology* 125 (1976): 79–82.

Meeker, C. Irving. "Use of Drugs and Intrauterine Devices for Birth Control." *New England Journal of Medicine* 280 (1969): 1058–60.

Mercer, Marilyn. "The Pill Can Change Your Diet Needs." *McCall's,* May 1972, 84.

Merlin, Donald H. *Pregnancy as a Disease: The Pill in Society.* Port Washington, N.Y.: Kennikat, 1976.

Merrill, L. Kent, Laurence I. Burd, and Daniel Ver Burg. "Laparoscopic Removal of Intraperitoneal Dalkon Shields: A Report of Three Cases." *American Journal of Obstetrics and Gynecology* 118 (1974): 1146–48.

Miller, George H. "IUD Expelled during Third Stage of Labor." *Obstetrics and Gynecology* 28 (1966): 877.

Mintz, Morton. *At Any Cost: Corporate Greed, Women, and the Dalkon Shield.* New York: Pantheon, 1985.

———. *The Pill: An Alarming Report.* Boston: Beacon, 1969.

———. *The Therapeutic Nightmare: A Report on Roles of the United States Food and Drug Administration, the American Medical Association, Pharmaceutical Manufacturers, and Others in Connection with Irrational and Massive Use of Prescription Drugs That May Be Worthless, Injurious or Even Lethal.* Boston: Houghton Mifflin, 1965.

Misenhimer, H. Robert, and Rafael Garcia-Bunuel. "Failure of Intrauterine Contraceptive Devices and Fungal Infection in the Fetus." *Obstetrics and Gynecology* 34 (1969): 368–72.

Mishell, Daniel R., Jr., Moustafa Aly El Habashy, Robert G. Good, and Dean L. Moyer. "Contraception with an Injectable Progestin: A Study of Its Use in Postpartum Women." *American Journal of Obstetrics and Gynecology* 101 (1968): 1046–53.

Mishell, Daniel R., Jr., Robert Israel, and Norman Fried. "A Study of the Copper T Intrauterine Contraceptive Device (TCu200) in Nulliparous Women." *American Journal of Obstetrics and Gynecology* 116 (1973): 1092–96.

Mishell, Daniel R., Jr., M. Talas, A. F. Parlow, and Dean L. Moyer. "Contraception by Means of a Silastic Vaginal Ring Impregnated With Medroxyprogesterone Acetate." *American Journal of Obstetrics and Gynecology* 107 (1970): 100–07.

Mohr, James C. *Abortion in America: The Origins and Evolution of National Policy, 1800–1900.* New York: Oxford University Press, 1978.

Moore, Emily. "To S. F.: My God, We've Been Telling You!" *Family Planning Perspectives* 4/1 (1972): 2–4.

"More Counterfeit Contraceptives." *FDA Consumer,* December 1985–January 1986, 3.

"More Than One Million Voluntary Sterilizations Performed in U.S. in 1980." *Family Planning Perspectives* 14/2 (1982): 99.

Morese, Kenneth N., William F. Peterson, and S. Thomas Allen. "Endometrial Effects of an Intrauterine Contraceptive Device." *Obstetrics and Gynecology* 28 (1966): 323–28.

Morgan, Susanne. *Coping with Hysterectomy: Your Own Choice, Your Own Solutions.* New York: Dial, 1982.

Morris, Naomi M., and J. Richard Udry. "Depression of Physical Activity by Contraceptive Pills." *American Journal of Obstetrics and Gynecology* 104 (1969): 1012–14.

Morris, W.I.C. "Tubal Ligation Failures." *The Lancet,* April 3, 1971, 706.

Morrison, Margaret. "Contraception with IUD's." *FDA Consumer,* February 1975, 15–20.

"Multiple Sclerosis—Effects of Spinal Anesthesia and Oral Contraceptives." *Journal of the American Medical Association* 212 (1970): 2129.

Nagel, Theodore C. "Intrauterine Contraceptive Devices: Complications Associated with Their Use." *Postgraduate Medicine* 73 (1983): 155–64.

Nakamoto, Masao, and Myron I. Buchman. "Complications of Intrauterine Contraceptive Devices: Report of 5 Cases of Ectopic Placement of Bow." *American Journal of Obstetrics and Gynecology* 94 (1966): 1073–78.

National Women's Health Network. *Depoprovera.* Washington: NWHN, 1985.

Nebel, William A., John L. Currie, and Richard E. Lassiter. "Clinical Experience with the Copper 7 Intrauterine Contraceptive Device: A Preliminary Report." *American Journal of Obstetrics and Gynecology* 126 (1976): 586–89.

Neutz, Eberhard, Arthur Silber, and Vincent J. Meredino. "Dalkon Shield Perforation of the Uterus and Urinary Bladder with Calculus Formation: Case Report." *American Journal of Obstetrics and Gynecology* 130 (1978): 848–49.

"The New Doubts about the Pill." *Life,* February 27, 1970, 28–29.

"A New Warning about Birth Control Pills." *Good Housekeeping,* August 1968, 156.

Newman, Lucile F. "Context Variables in Fertility Regulation." In *Women's Medicine,* ed. Lucile F. Newman, 179–92. New Brunswick: Rutgers University Press, 1985.

———. "An Introduction to Population Anthropology." In *Women's Medicine,* ed. Lucile F. Newman, 1–24. New Brunswick: Rutgers University Press, 1985.

———, ed. *Women's Medicine: A Cross-Cultural Study of Indigenous Fertility Regulation.* New Brunswick: Rutgers University Press, 1985.

Newton, John, Julian Elias, and Anthony Johnson. "Immediate Post-Termination Insertion of Copper 7 and Dalkon Shield Intrauterine Contraceptive Devices." *Journal of Obstetrics and Gynecology of the British Commonwealth* 81 (1974): 389–92.

Ngin, Choi-Swanj. "Indigenous Fertility Regulating Methods among Two Chinese Communities in Malaysia." In *Women's Medicine,* ed. Lucile F. Newman, 25–42. New Brunswick: Rutgers University Press, 1985.

Nilsson, Carl Gustaf, Pertti L. A. Lahteenmaki, and Dale N. Robertson. "Sustained Intrauterine Release of Levonorgestrel over Five Years." *Fertility and Sterility* 45 (1986): 805–07.

Nilsson, O., and Kerstin Hagenfeldt. "Scanning Electron Microscopy of Human Uterine Epithelium Influenced by the TCu Intrauterine Contraceptive Device." *American Journal of Obstetrics and Gynecology* 117 (1973): 469–72.

"Now! Something Better Than . . . 'The Pill'?" *McCall's,* February 1965, 42.

Nygren, Karl-Gosta, and Elof D. B. Johansen. "Premature Onset of Menstrual Bleeding during Ovulatory Cycles in Women with an Intrauterine Contraceptive Device." *American Journal of Obstetrics and Gynecology* 117 (1973): 971–75.

Ober, William B., Aquiles J. Sobrero, and Ada B. de Chalon. "Endometrial Findings after Insertion of Stainless Steel Spring IUD." *Obstetrics and Gynecology* 36 (1970): 62–69.

Ober, William B., Aquiles J. Sobrero, Ada B. de Chalon, and Jon Goodman. "Polyethylene Intrauterine Contraceptive Device: Endometrial Changes Following Long-Term Use." *Journal of the American Medical Association* 212 (1976): 765–69.

Ober, William B., Aquiles J. Sobrero, Robert Kurman, and Saul Gold. "Endometrial Emorphology and Polyethylene Intrauterine Devices: A Study of 200 Endometrial Biopsies." *Obstetrics and Gynecology* 32 (1968): 782–93.

O'Brien, Paul K. "Abdominal and Endometrial Actinomycosis Associated with an Intrauterine Device." *Canadian Medical Association Journal* 112 (1975): 596–97.

Olsson, Sven-Eric, Viveca Odlind, Elof D. B. Johansson, and Marie-Louise Nordstrom. "Plasma Levels of Levonorgestrel and Free Levonorgestrel Index in Women Using Norplant Implants or Two Covered Rods (Norplant-2)." *Contraception* 35 (1987): 215–28.

"Oral Contraceptive Effects on the Breast." *Journal of the American Medical Association* 224 (1973): 249, col. 3.

"Oral Contraceptives: Balancing Risks against Benefits." *Science News* 95 (1969): 42.

"Oral Contraceptives: Only a Yellow Light." *Science News* 96 (1969): 198.

"Oral Contraceptives May Complicate Fight with VD." *Journal of the American Medical Association* 216 (1971): 1546.

"Oral Contraceptives May Tend to Protect against Benign Breast Cancer." *Journal of the American Medical Association* 217 (1971): 20–21.

Ory, Howard W. "The Noncontraceptive Benefits from Oral Contraceptive Use." *Family Planning Perspectives* 14/4 (1982): 182–84.

———. "A Review of the Association between Intrauterine Devices and Acute Pelvic Inflammatory Disease." *Journal of Reproductive Medicine* 20 (1978): 200–204.

Ory, Howard W., and the Women's Health Study. "Ectopic Pregnancy and Intrauterine Contraceptive Devices: New Perspectives." *Obstetrics and Gynecology* 57 (1981): 137–43.

Osler, Mogens, and Paul E. Lebech. "A New Form of Intrauterine Contraceptive Device." *American Journal of Obstetrics and Gynecology* 102 (1968): 1173–76.

Oster, Gerald, and Miklos P. Salgo. "The Copper Intrauterine Device and Its Mode of Action." *New England Journal of Medicine* 293 (1975): 432–38.

Ostergard, Donald R. "Intrauterine Contraception in Multiparas with the Dalkon Shield." *American Journal of Obstetrics and Gynecology* 119 (1974): 1022–37.

———. "Intrauterine Contraception in Nulliparas with the Dalkon Shield." *American Journal of Obstetrics and Gynecology* 116 (1973): 1088–91.

Ostrander, Sheila, and Lynn Schroeder. "Birth Control By Astrology? A European Doctor's Controversial Theory about Fertility in Women." *McCall's,* May 1972, 84–88.

"Our Readers Talk Back about the Birth Control Pills." *Ladies' Home Journal,* November 1967, 92.

Pardthaisong, Tieng. "Return of Fertility after Use of the Injectable Contraceptive Depo Provera: Up-Dated Data Analysis." *Journal of Biosocial Science* 16 (1984): 23–34.

Patchell, R. D. "Rectouterine Fistula Associated with the Cu-7 Intrauterine Contraceptive Device." *American Journal of Obstetrics and Gynecology* 126 (1976): 292–93.

"Patient Labeling Now Required for IUD's." *FDA Consumer,* December 1977, 5.

Paul, Eve W. "Population Law or Women's Health Law?" *Family Planning Perspectives* 14/6 (1982): 292.

Peel, John, and Griselda Carr. *Contraception and Family Design: A Study of Birth Planning in Contemporary Society.* New York: Longmans, 1975.

"Pelvic Inflammatory Disease among Dalkon Shield Users." *Journal of the American Medical Association* 249 (1983): 2757.

"Pelvic Inflammatory Disease and the Dalkon Shield." *Obstetrics and Gynecology* 64 (1984): 297–300.

Pena, Eduardo F. "Perforation of Rectovaginal Septum by Intrauterine Device." *Obstetrics and Gynecology* 28 (1966): 731.

Peplow, Victor, William G. Breed, and Peter Eckstein. "Studies in Uterine Flushings in the Baboon: II. The Effect of an Intrauterine Contraceptive Device in Certain Biochemical Parameters." *American Journal of Obstetrics and Gynecology* 116 (1973): 780–84.

"Perforation Risk Greater When IUD's Are Inserted in Breastfeeding Women." *International Family Planning Perspectives* 9 (1983): 24.

Perlmutter, Johanna F. "Experience with the Dalkon Shield as a Contraceptive Device." *Obstetrics and Gynecology* 43 (1974): 443–46.

Perry, Susan, and Jim Dawson. *Nightmare: Women and the Dalkon Shield.* New York: Macmillan, 1985.

Persson, Elisabeth, and Kenneth Holmberg. "Genital Colonization by Actinomyces Israelii and Serologic Immune Response to the Bacterium after Five Years Use of the Same Copper Intra-Uterine Device." *Acta Obstetricia Gynecologica Scandinavica* 63 (1984): 203–05.

Persson, Elisabeth, Kenneth Holmberg, S. Dahlgren, and L. Nilsson. "Actinomyces Israelii in the Genital Tract of Women with and without Intra-Uterine Contraceptive Devices." *Acta Obstetricia Gynecologica Scandinavica* 62 (1983): 563–68.

" 'The Pill.' " *FDA Consumer,* December 1972–January 1973, 16–18.

"The Pill: Cloudy Verdict." *Newsweek,* September 15, 1969, 90.

"The Pill and Cancer." *Newsweek,* August 11, 1969, 59.

"Pill and IUD Use at PPFA Clinics Decline, Diaphragm Use Rises." *Family Planning Perspectives* 14/3 (1982): 152.

"Pill Does Not Increase Risk of Breast Cancer Even after Years of Use." *Family Planning Perspectives* 14/4 (1982): 216–20.

" 'The Pill' for Men?" *Newsweek,* July 14, 1969, 62.

"The Pill Goes to Washington." *Business Week,* January 10, 1970, 31–32.

"The Pill Is Hard to Follow." *Business Week,* January 31, 1970, 80.

"The 'Pill' May Inhibit Early Cancer, Study Suggests." *Journal of the American Medical Association* 220 (1972): 775–77.

"The Pill on Trial." *Time,* January 26, 1970, 60–62.

"The Pill Trial *(contd.).*" *Time,* March 9, 1970, 32.

"Pill Users Protected against V/D If They Have Used OCs for Longer Than One Year." *Family Planning Perspectives* 14/1 (1982): 32–33.

Pincus, G. *The Control of Fertility.* New York: Academic, 1965.

Piner, M. Steven, John P. Whiteley, and Ronald J. Bologuese. "Effect of an Intrauterine

Contraceptive Device upon Cervical and Endometrial Exfoliative Cytology." *Obstetrics and Gynecology* 28 (1966): 528–31.

Poland, Betty J., and Katherine A. Ash. "The Influence of Recent Use of an Oral Contraceptive on Early Intrauterine Development." *American Journal of Obstetrics and Gynecology* 116 (1973): 1138–42.

Pollock, Mary. "Letting Intrauterine Devices Lie." *British Medical Journal* 285 (1982): 1049.

Population Crisis Committee. *Population Research.* Washington: PCC, 1971.

Potts, Malcolm, and John M. Paxman. "Depo-Provera: Ethical Issues in Its Testing and Distribution." *Journal of Medical Ethics* (1984): 9–20.

Powell, L. C., Jr., and R. J. Seymour. "Effects of Depo-Medroxyprogesterone Acetate as a Contraceptive Agent." *American Journal of Obstetrics and Gynecology* 110 (1971): 36–41.

"A Pox on the Pill." *Journal of the American Medical Association* 213 (1970): 1481.

"PPFA Clinics Advised: Remove Dalkon Shields, Prescribe Low-Dose Pill." *Family Planning Perspectives* 16/5 (1984): 237–38.

"Pregnancy and 'Pill' Can Lead to Liver Ailment." *Journal of the American Medical Association* 212 (1976): 2046.

Preston, S. N. "The Oral Contraceptive Controversy." *American Journal of Obstetrics and Gynecology* 111 (1971): 994–1006.

"The Pros and Cons of the Pill." *Time,* May 2, 1969, 58.

"Proselytizers for Prophylactics." *Time,* December 7, 1970, 98–99.

"Ralph Nader Reports [on DES]." *Ladies' Home Journal,* August 1973.

Raspe, Gerhard, and S. Bernhar, eds. *Advances in the Biosciences, 10. Schering Workshop on Contraception: The Masculine Gender—Berlin, November 29 to December 2, 1972.* Oxford: Pergamon, 1973.

"Recalling a Pill." *Time,* February 9, 1970, 39.

Reed, James. *From Private Vice to Public Virtue: The Birth Control Movement and American Society since 1830.* New York: Basic Books, 1978.

"Re-evaluating the Pill." *Newsweek,* January 12, 1970, 66.

"Reports Conflict on Link between Hysterectomy, Prior Tubal Sterilization." *Family Planning Perspectives* 15/5 (1983): 229–30.

Reynolds, C. "Toxic Shock Syndrome Associated with a Contraceptive Diaphragm." *Canadian Medical Association Journal* 128 (1983): 1144.

"The Rhythm Method of Birth Control." *America,* June 7, 1969, 663.

Rifai, Samy F. "A New Contraceptive Device with Reduced Expulsion Rate." *American Journal of Obstetrics and Gynecology* 104 (1969): 1113–17.

Rifkin, Ira, Lila E. Nachtigall, and E. Mark Beckman. "Amenorrhea Following Use of Oral Contraceptives." *American Journal of Obstetrics and Gynecology* 113 (1972): 420–31.

"Right Now: Scorecard on Birth Control." *McCall's,* November 1973, 47.

"Risk of Menstrual Problems Increased among Women Sterilized before 1975." *Family Planning Perspectives* 17/6 (1985): 272–74.

"Risk of Pelvic Infection Associated with Intrauterine Devices." *British Medical Journal* (1976): 717–18.

"Risk of PID 5X Greater from Dalkon Shield Than from Other IUD's." *Family Planning Perspectives* 15/5 (1983): 225.

"Risk of Tubal Infection from Chlamydial PID Reduced by Pill Use." *Family Planning Perspectives* 17/6 (1985): 269–70.

"Risks from Dalkon Shield." *FDA Consumer,* May 1985, 35.

Rivera, Roberto, Jose R. Gaitan, Martha Ortega, Consuelo Flores, and Ana Hernandez. "The Use of Biodegradable Norethiserone Implants as a 6-month Contraceptive System." *Fertility and Sterility* 42 (1984): 228–32.

Roberts, Daniel K., Douglas V. Horbelt, and Nola J. Walker. "Scanning Electron Microscopy of the Multifilament IUD String." *Contraception* 29 (1984): 215–29.

Roberts, Helen. *Doing Feminist Research.* London: Routledge and Kegan Paul, 1981.

Roberts, James M., and William J. Ledger. "Operative Removal of Intraperitoneal Intrauterine Contraceptive Devices—A Reappraisal." *American Journal of Obstetrics and Gynecology* 112 (1972): 863–65.

Robin, Eugene Debs. *Matters of Life and Death: Risks vs. Benefits of Medical Care.* New York: W.H. Treimer, 1984.

"Robins' Dalkon Shield Found No More Risky Than Other IUDs." *Wall Street Journal,* October 14, 1974, 2.

"Robins Warns That Its IUD May Cause Severe Complications, Including Death." *Wall Street Journal,* May 30, 1974, 8.

Robins, Joel, Lloyd Mitler, Lorey Pollack, and Leon I. Mann. "Difficult Elective Removal of a Majzlin Spring Intrauterine Device." *Journal of Reproductive Medicine* 14 (1975): 68–69.

Robinson, S. C. "Pregnancy Outcome Following Oral Contraceptives." *American Journal of Obstetrics and Gynecology* 109 (1971): 354–68.

Rock, John. "The Significance of Population Research." In *Population Research.* Washington: Population Crisis Council, 1971.

Rooks, Judith P. "Informing Providers, Informing Users." *Family Planning Perspectives* 15/6 (1983): 295–97.

———. "The Feminist Health Book: *The New Our Bodies, Ourselves: A Book by and for Women.*" *Family Planning Perspectives* 17/5 (1985): 209–15.

Rosado, A., Juan Jose Hicks, R. Aznar, and J. Martinez-Mavauton. "Effect of the Intrauterine Contraceptive Device upon the Biochemical Composition of Human Endometrium." *American Journal of Obstetrics and Gynecology* 114 (1972): 88–92.

Rosenberg, Max. "Factors in Oral Contraception Related Hypertension." *American Journal of Obstetrics and Gynecology* 104 (1969): 1221–22.

Rosenberg, Michael J., Peter M. Layde, Howard W. Ory, Lilo T. Strauss, Judith Bourne Rooks, and George L. Rubin. "Agreement between Women's Histories of Oral Contraceptives Use and Physician Records." *International Journal of Epidemiology* 12 (1983): 84–87.

Rovinsky, Joseph J. "Clinical Effectiveness of a Contraceptive Cream." *Obstetrics and Gynecology* 23 (1964): 125–31.

Rowland, Thomas C., Jr. "Severe Peritonitis Complicating an Intrauterine Contraceptive Device." *American Journal of Obstetrics and Gynecology* 110 (1971): 786–87.

Roy, Subir, Donna Cooper, and Daniel R. Mishell, Jr. "Experience with Three Different Models for the Copper T Intrauterine Contraceptive Device in Nulliparous Women." *American Journal of Obstetrics and Gynecology* 119 (1974): 414–17.

Rozin, Samuel, and Amiram Adoni. "A New Intrauterine Contraceptive Device: An Open Ring." *Obstetrics and Gynecology* 36 (1970): 304–05.

Ruben, George L., Howard W. Ory, and Peter M. Layde. "Oral Contraceptives and Pelvic Inflammatory Disease." *American Journal of Obstetrics and Gynecology* 144 (1982): 630–35.

Salaverry, G., M. Del C. Mendez, J. Zipper, and M. Medel. "Copper Determination and Localization in Different Morphologic Components of Human Endometrium during the Menstrual Cycle in Copper Intrauterine Contraceptive Device Wearers." *American Journal of Obstetrics and Gynecology* 115 (1973): 163–68.

Salhanick, Hilton A., and David A. Kinnis. *Metabolic Effects of Gonadal Hormones and Contraceptive Steroids.* New York: Plenum, 1969.

Sammour, M. B., S. G. Iskander, and S. F. Rifai. "Combined Histologic and Cytologic Study of Intrauterine Contraception." *American Journal of Obstetrics and Gynecology* 98 (1967): 946–55.

Sanchez, V. Diaz, J. Garza Flores, S. Jiminez-Thomas, and H. W. Rudel. "Development of a Low-Dose Monthly Injectable Contraceptive System: Pharmaceutic and Pharmacodynamic Studies." *Contraception* 35 (1987): 57–67.

Savage, Wendy. "Is the Dalkon Shield More Dangerous Than Other IUCD's?" *British Medical Journal* 291 (1985): 345.

Schmidt, Waldemar A. "IUDs, Inflammation, and Infection: Assessment after Two Decades of IUD Use." *Human Pathology* 13 (1982): 878–81.

Scholl, Theresa O., Eugene Sobel, Koray Tanfer, Ellen Soefer, and Bruce Sardman. "Effects of Vaginal Spermicides on Pregnancy Outcome." *Family Planning Perspectives* 15/5 (1983): 244.

Schwan, Anna, Tom Ahren, and Arne Victor. "Effects of Contraceptive Vaginal Ring Treatment on Vaginal Bacteriology and Cytology." *Contraception* 28 (1983): 347–49.

Schweid, Abraham K., and G. Bruce Hopkins. "Monilial Chorionitis Associated with an Intrauterine Contraceptive Device." *Obstetrics and Gynecology* 31 (1968): 719–21.

Scott, Roger B. "Critical Illnesses and Deaths Associated with Intrauterine Devices." *Obstetrics and Gynecology* 31 (1968): 322–27.

Scott, William C. "Pelvic Abscesses in Association with Intrauterine Contraceptive Device." *American Journal of Obstetrics and Gynecology* 131 (1978): 149–56.

Scully, Diane. *Men Who Control Women's Health: The Miseducation of Obstetrician-Gynecologists.* Boston: Houghton Mifflin, 1980.

Seaman, Barbara. *The Doctors' Case against the Pill.* Rev. ed. Garden City, N.Y.: Doubleday, 1980.

———. "Tell Me Doctor: 'Why Did Birth Control Fail Me?'" *Ladies' Home Journal,* November 1965, 166–67.

Seaman, Barbara, and Gideon Seaman. *Women and the Crisis in Sex Hormones.* New York: Bantam, 1978.

"The Search for a Birth Control Method to Replace The Pill." *Good Housekeeping,* September 1967, 179–81.

Sedlis, Alexander, and J. Victor Reyniah. "Endometrial Leukocytes in Patients Using Intrauterine Contraceptive Devices." *American Journal of Obstetrics and Gynecology,* 108 (1970): 1209–12.

Segall, M. *Pharmaceuticals and Health Planning in Developing Countries.* Brighton: Institute for Development Studies at Sussex, 1975.

Seward, Paul N., Robert Israel, and Charles A. Ballard. "Ectopic Pregnancy and Intrauterine Contraception: A Definite Relationship." *Obstetrics and Gynecology* 40 (1972): 214–16.

"Sexuality: Changing Standards." *Time,* May 16, 1969, 52.

Seymour, R. J., and L. C. Powell, Jr. "Depo-Medroxyprogesterone Acetate as a Contraceptive." *Obstetrics and Gynecology* 36 (1970): 589–96.

Shaaban, M. M., and M. Salah. "A Two-Year Experience With Norplant® Implants in Assiut, Egypt." *Contraception* 29 (1984): 335–43.

Shaila, Nariyondada, Mary E. Lane, and Aquiles J. Sobrero. "A Comparative Randomized Double-Blind Study of the Copper T200 and Copper 7 Intrauterine Contraceptive Devices with Modified Insertion Techniques." *American Journal of Obstetrics and Gynecology* 120 (1974): 110–15.

Shainwald, Sybil. "RX for Your Legal Health: Medical Malpractice 'Crisis'?" *Network News,* January–February 1987, 5.

————. "The Story of the Dalkon Shield." *The Dalkon Shield.* Washington: NWHN, 1985.

————, ed. *The Dalkon Shield.* Washington: NWHN, 1985.

Shanly, Sven Olaf, Lasi Molsted-Pedersen, and Ahti Kosonen. "Consequences of Intrauterine Contraception in Diabetic Women." *Fertility and Sterility* 42 (1984): 568–72.

Shapiro, Howard I. *The Birth Control Book.* New York: St. Martin's, 1977.

Sheffield, William H., Samuel D. Soule, and Gudofredo M. Herzog. "Cyclic Endometrial Changes in Response to Monthly Injections of an Estrogen-Progestogen Contraceptive Drug: A Histologic Study." *American Journal of Obstetrics and Gynecology* 103 (1969): 828–35.

Sherrod, Dale B., and Willard Nicholl. "Electrocardiographic Changes during Intrauterine Contraceptive Device Insertion." *American Journal of Obstetrics and Gynecology* 119 (1974): 1044–51.

Shine, Robert M., and Joseph F. Thompson. "The in Situ IUD and Pregnancy Outcome." *American Journal of Obstetrics and Gynecology* 119 (1974): 124–30.

Shirley, Robert L. "The Dalkon Shield in Private Practice: A Disappointment." *American Journal of Obstetrics and Gynecology* 121 (1975): 564–65.

Shrogie, John J. "Clinical Safety of Oral Contraceptives." *FDA Papers,* June 1969, 4.

Siegler, Alvin M. "Removal of Ectopic Intrauterine Contraceptive Devices Aided by Laparoscopy: A Report of 3 Cases and a Review of the Literature." *American Journal of Obstetrics and Gynecology* 115 (1973): 158–62.

Siegler, Alvin M., and Chi Huei Chen. "Uterine Perforation during Removal of a Broken Majzlin Spring." *Fertility and Sterility* 23 (1972): 776–78.

Siegler, Alvin M., and Louis M. Hellman. "The Effect of the Intrauterine Contraceptive Coil on the Oviduct." *Obstetrics and Gynecology* 23 (1964): 173–75.

Silberman, Eugene, Martin L. Stone, and Elizabeth B. Connell. "The 'M,' a New Intrauterine Contraceptive Device." *American Journal of Obstetrics and Gynecology* 105 (1969): 279–81.

Silverman, Milton. *The Drugging of the Americas.* Berkeley: University of California Press, 1976.

————. "The Epidemiology of Drug Promotion." *International Journal of Health Services* 7 (1977): 157–66.

Silverman, Milton, and Philip R. Lee. *Pills, Profits, and Politics.* Berkeley: University of California Press, 1974.

Silverman, Milton, and Mia Lydecker. *Prescription for Death: The Drugging of the Third World.* Berkeley: University of California Press, 1982.

"A Simple Way to Remove IUDs after Perforation." *Journal of the American Medical Association* 220 (1972): 781–84.

Sivin, Irving, Francisco Alvarez Sanchez, Solidad Diaz, Pentti Holma, Elsimar Coutinho, Olivia McDonald, Dale N. Robertson, and Janet Stern. "Three-Year Experience with Norplant Subdermal Contraception." *Fertility and Sterility* 39 (1983): 799–808.

Sivin, Irving, Janet Stern, Juan Diaz, Anibal Faundes, Sayed El Mahgoub, Solidad Diaz, Margarita Parez, Elsimar Coutinho, Carlos E. R. Mattos, Terry McCarthy, D. R. Mishell, Jr., Donna Shoyse, Francisco Alvarez Sanchez, Vivian Brache, and Elvira Jimenez. "21 Years of Intrauterine Contraception with Levonorgestral and with Copper: A Randomized Comparison of the TCu 380 Ag and Levonorgestral 20 MCG/Day Devices." *Contraception* 35 (1987): 245–55.

Slaughter, Laura, and David J. Morris. "Peritoneal-Cutaneous Fistula Secondary to a Perforated Dalkon Shield." *American Journal of Obstetrics and Gynecology* 124 (1976): 206–07.

Smith, M., and P. Blais. "Preliminary Findings on Used Cervical Caps." *Contraception* 29 (1984): 527–32.

Smith, May, and B. Norman Barwin. "Vaginal Mechanical Contraceptive Devices." *Canadian Medical Association Journal* 129 (1983): 699–701.

Smith, P. A., C. J. Ellis, R. A. Sparks, and J. Guillebaud. "Deaths Associated with Intrauterine Contraceptive Devices in the United Kingdom between 1973 and 1983." *British Medical Journal* 287 (1983): 1537–38.

Smith, Ronald W. "Hypertension and Oral Contraceptives." *American Journal of Obstetrics and Gynecology* 113 (1972): 482–87.

Snowden, R., and B. Pearson. "Pelvic Infection: A Comparison of the Dalkon Shield and Three Other Intrauterine Devices." *British Medical Journal* 288 (1984): 1570–73.

Sobrero, Aquiles J., and Daniel Pierotti. "Majzlin Intrauterine Contraceptive Spring: Report of a Clinical Study." *Obstetrics and Gynecology* 36 (1970): 911–18.

Soichet, Samuel. "Ypsilon: A New Silicone-Covered Stainless Steel Intrauterine Contraceptive Device." *American Journal of Obstetrics and Gynecology* 114 (1972): 938–41.

Solish, George I., Schuyler G. Kohl, and Gregory Majzlin. "Effectiveness of the Majzlin Spring Intrauterine Contraceptive Device." *American Journal of Obstetrics and Gynecology* 114 (1972): 106–11.

Solish, George I., and Gregory Majzlin. "New Stainless Steel Spring for Intrauterine Contraception." *Obstetrics and Gynecology* 32 (1968): 116–19.

Southam, Anna L. "What's New in Family Planning." *Parents Magazine,* November 1965.

Sparks, R. A. "Endocarditis and the Intrauterine Device." *The Lancet,* April 28, 1984, 957.

"Special Report Based on New Medical Evidence: Must We Now Ban the Birth Control Pills?" *Good Housekeeping,* February 1966, 67–70.

Spitz, Irving M. "Antiprogestins: Prospects for a Once-a-Month Pill." *Family Planning Perspectives* 17/6 (1985): 260–62.

"Sponge for Contraception." *FDA Consumer,* July–August 1983, 3.

Sprague, Arnold D., and Van R. Jenkins II. "Perforation of the Uterus with a Shield Intrauterine Device." *Obstetrics and Gynecology* 41 (1973): 80–82.

Stacey, Judith. "Are Feminists Afraid to Leave Home? The Challenge of Conservative Pro-Family Feminism." In *What Is Feminism? A Re-Examination,* ed. Juliet Mitchell and Ann Oakley, 208–37. New York: Pantheon, 1986.

Stadel, Bruce V., and Sarah Schlesselman. "Extent of Surgery for Pelvic Inflammatory Disease in Relation to Duration of Intrauterine Device Use." *Obstetrics and Gynecology* 63 (1984): 171–77.

Starr, Paul. *The Social Transformation of American Medicine.* New York: Basic Books, 1982.

"Sterilizations Off Sharply in 1982: Drop Due Mostly to Vasectomy Decline." *Family Planning Perspectives* 16/1 (1984): 40–41.

Stewart, Elizabeth. "Mechanical Methods of Contraception." *The Practitioner* 205 (1970): 13–19.

Stokes, Bruce. *Men and Family Planning: Worldwatch Paper 41.* Washington: Worldwatch Institute, 1980.

Strauss, Anselm L. *Qualitative Analysis for Social Scientists.* New York: Cambridge University Press, 1987.

"Study Examines Ectopic Pregnancy Risk after Completed Childbearing." *Family Planning Perspectives* 14/6 (1982): 336–37.

"Study of Some 20,000 Men Finds No Evidence Vasectomy Has Any Adverse Health Consequences." *Family Planning Perspectives* 16/1 (1984): 35–36.

"Study Results Cast Doubt on Pill-Hypertension Link." *Journal of the American Medical Association* 228 (1974): 1507–08.

Sukkary-Stolba, Soheir. "Indigenous Fertility Regulating Methods in Two Egyptian Villages." In *Women's Medicine: A Cross-Cultural Study of Indigenous Fertility Regulation,* ed. Lucile F. Newman. New Brunswick: Rutgers University Press, 1985.

Sung, Shih, Qian Li-Jian, and Liu Xuan. "Comparative Clinical Experience with 3 IUDs, TCu 380 Ag, TCu 220C and Mahua Ring, in Tianjin, People's Republic of China." *Contraception* 29 (1984): 229–39.

Sweet, Ellen. "A Failed 'Revolution.' " *Ms.,* March 1988, 75–78.

Svenson, Lars, Lars Westrom, and Per-Anders Mardh. "Contraceptives and Acute Salpingitis." *Journal of the American Medical Association* 251 (1984): 2553–55.

Swerdloff, Ronald S., David J. Handelsman, and Shalender Bhasin. "Hormonal Effects of GnRH Agonist in the Human Male: An Approach to Male Contraception Using Combined Androgen and GnRH Agonist Treatment." *Journal of Steroid Biochemistry* 23 (1985): 855–61.

Tadese, E., and K. Hamstiker. "Evaluation of 24 Patients with IUD-Related Problems: Hysteroscopic Findings." *European Journal of Obstetrics, Gynecology, and Reproductive Biology* (1985): 37–41.

"Take Out Dalkon Shield." *FDA Consumer,* February 1985, 37.

Targum, Steven D., and Nicholas H. Wright. "Association of the Intrauterine Device and Pelvic Inflammatory Disease: A Retrospective Pilot Study." *American Journal of Epidemiology* 100 (1974): 262–71.

Tatum, Howard J. "Intrauterine Contraception." *American Journal of Obstetrics and Gynecology* 112 (1972): 1000–23.

————. "Metallic Copper as an Intrauterine Contraceptive Agent." *American Journal of Obstetrics and Gynecology* 117 (1973): 602–19.

————. "Milestones in Intrauterine Device Development." *Fertility and Sterility* 39 (1983): 141–43.

Tatum, Howard J., and Elizabeth B. Connell. "A Decade of Intrauterine Contraception: 1976 to 1986." *Fertility and Sterility* 46 (1986): 173–92.

Tatum, Howard J., Elsimar M. Coutinho, J. Adeodato Filho, and Ana Rita S. Sant'Anna. "Acceptability of Long-Term Contraceptive Steroid Administration in Humans by Subcutaneous Silastic Capsules." *American Journal of Obstetrics and Gynecology* 105 (1969): 1139–43.

Tatum, Howard J., Frederick H. Schmidt, David Phillips, Maclyn McCarty, and William O'Leary. "The Dalkon Shield Controversy: Structural and Bacteriological Studies of IUD Tails." *Journal of the American Medical Association* 231 (1975): 711–17.

Taylor, E. Stewart, James H. McMillan, Benjamin E. Greer, William Droegemueller, and Horace E. Thompson. "The Intrauterine Device and Tubo-ovarian Abscess." *American Journal of Obstetrics and Gynecology* 123 (1975): 338–48.

Taylor, Marshall B., and Martin B. Kass. "Effect of Oral Contraception on Glucose Metabolism." *American Journal of Obstetrics and Gynecology* 102 (1968): 1035–38

Taylor, Thomas E. "Extremity Red Streaks and the Pill—Lymphangitis or Thrombophlebitis?" *Journal of the American Medical Association* 215 (1971): 1164.

Taylor, Walter W., Francis G. Martin, Signe A. Pritchard, and Jack A. Pritchard. "Complications from Majzlin Spring Intrauterine Devices." *Obstetrics and Gynecology* 41 (1973): 404–12.

Tejuja, Sahita, and Parvati K. Malkani. "Clinical Significance of Correlation between Size of Uterine Cavity and I.U.C.D.: A Study by Planimeter-Hysterogram Technique." *American Journal of Obstetrics and Gynecology* 105 (1969): 620–27.

Templeton, J. S. "Clinical Experience with the Dalkon Shield." *British Medical Journal,* September 8, 1973, 542.

————. "Septic Abortion and the Dalkon Shield." *British Medical Journal,* June 15, 1974, 612.

"Thalidomide Sequel." *Time,* February 9, 1970, 29.

Thompson, Richard C. "A 'Complaint Department' for Medical Devices." *FDA Consumer,* March 1987, 10–13.

Thomsen, Russell J. "Inflammatory Reaction to the Dalkon Shield." *Obstetrics and Gynecology* 46 (1975): 116.

————. "Pregnancy in the Presence of an Intrauterine Contraceptive Device and Amniotic Fluid Embolism: A Possible Association." *American Journal of Obstetrics and Gynecology* 121 (1975): 279–81.

Thomsen, Russell J., Sam Pasquale, and John Nosher. "Ultrasonic Visualization of Norplant Subdermal Contraceptive Devices." *International Journal of Gynecology and Obstetrics* 23 (1985): 223–27.

Tichauer, Ruth W., and Gaston Maure. "Increasing Consumer Participation in Professional Goal Setting: Contraception and Therapeutic Abortion." *Journal of American Medical Women's Association* 27 (1972): 365–75.

Tietze, Christopher. "Contraception with Intrauterine Devices: 1959–1966." *American Journal of Obstetrics and Gynecology* 96 (1966): 1043–54.

Tietze, Christopher, and Sara Lewit, eds. *Intra-Uterine Contraceptive Devices: Proceedings of the Conference, April 30–May 1, 1962, New York City.* International Congress Series No. 54. New York: Excerpts Medica Foundation, 1962.

"Toxic Shock Syndrome and the Vaginal Contraceptive Sponge." *Journal of the American Medical Association* 251 (1985): 1015–16.

"Troubles with I.U.C.D.s" *British Medical Journal,* April 1973, 2–3.

"Two Apostles of Control." *Life,* April 17, 1970, 32–37.

"Two Studies Find No Link between Use of Oral Contraceptives and Development of Pituitary Tumors." *Family Planning Perspectives* 15/6 (1983): 283–84.

Tyler, Carl W., Jr. "Planned Parenthood: Ideas for the 1980s." *Family Planning Perspectives* 14/4 (1982): 221–23.

Tyler, Edward T. "How Soon Will We Have the 'Ideal' Contraceptive?" *Journal of the American Medical Association* 219 (1972): 1333.

Tyson, J.E.A. "Oral Contraception and Elevated Blood Pressure." *American Journal of Obstetrics and Gynecology* 100 (1968): 875–76.

Udry, J. Richard, Lydia T. Clark, Charles L. Chase, and Marvin Levy. "Can Mass Media Advertising Increase Contraceptive Use?" *Family Planning Perspectives* 4/3 (1972): 37–44.

U.S. Congress. House. Select Committee on Population. *The Depo-Provera Debate,* 95th Cong., 2d sess., 1978.

———. Senate. Select Committee on Small Business. Subcommittee on Monopoly. *Present Status of Competition in the Pharmaceutical Industry.* 91st Cong., 2d sess., 1970. Document No. 40-471-70.

U.S. Food and Drug Administration. Advisory Committee on Obstetrics and Gynecology. *Report on Intrauterine Contraceptive Devices.* 1968. Document No. 29-137 0-68-3.

———. *Report on Oral Contraceptives.* 1966. Document No. 228-677-66-2.

———. *Second Report on Intrauterine Devices.* 1979. Document No. 017-012-00276-5.

———. *Second Report on Oral Contraceptives.* August 1, 1969. Document No. 362-666-0-69-2.

"Vasectomy: Little Effect on Men's Blood Pressure or Blood Composition." *Family Planning Perspectives* 14/4 (1982): 212–13.

Vaughan, Paul. *The Pill on Trial.* New York: Coward-McCann, 1970.

Vessey, M. P., D. Yeates, Rosemary Flanel, and Kim McPherson. "Pelvic Inflammatory Disease and the Intrauterine Device: Findings in a Large Cohort Study." *British Medical Journal* 282 (1981): 855–57.

Vessey, M. P., M. Lawless, Kim McPherson, and D. Yeates. "Fertility after Stopping Use of Intrauterine Contraceptive Devices." *British Medical Journal* 286 (1983): 106.

Viechnicki, M. Bruce. "Septicemia and Abortion with the Cu-7." *American Journal of Obstetrics and Gynecology* 129 (1977): 203–30.

"Virtually Failsafe IUD Seen in Year." *Journal of the American Medical Association* 212 (1970): 1136–37.

Wade, Priscilla H. "Why I'll Give My Daughter the Pill." *Redbook,* June 1970, 30.

Walker, Alice. "The Abortion." In *You Can't Keep a Good Woman Down: Stories by Alice Walker,* ed. Alice Walker, 64–76. New York: Harcourt Brace Jovanovich, 1980.

Ward, Martha C. *Poor Women, Powerful Men: America's Great Experiment in Family Planning.* Boulder, Colo.: Westview, 1986.

Wasserthal-Smoller, Sylvia, Charles B. Arnold, Raymond C. Lerner, and Susan L. Heim-
    rath. "Contraceptive Practices of Wives of Obstetricians." *American Journal of
    Obstetrics and Gynecology* 117 (1973): 709–15.
Weekes, Leroy R. "Complications of Intrauterine Contraceptive Devices." *Journal of the
    National Medical Association* 67 (1975): 1–10.
Weinberg, Roy David. *Family Planning and the Law.* Dobbs Ferry, N.Y.: Oceana, 1979.
————. *Laws Governing Family Planning.* Dobbs Ferry, N.Y.: Oceana, 1968.
Weinstein, Bette. "Birth Control Pill for Men." *McCall's,* July 1974, 34–35.
Weisberg, Edith, and Ian S. Fraser. "Fertility Following Reversal of Male and Female
    Sterilization." *Contraception* 26 (1982): 361–69.
Weiss, Barry D. "The Majzlin Spring Revisited." *American Family Practitioner* 26 (1982):
    123–24.
Westoff, Charles F. "The Modernization of U.S. Contraceptive Practice." *Family Planning
    Perspectives* 4/3 (1972): 9–12.
Westoff, Charles F., and Norman B. Ryder. *The Contraceptive Revolution.* Princeton: Prince-
    ton University Press, 1977.
Westrom, Lars. "Effect of Acute Pelvic Inflammatory Disease on Fertility." *American
    Journal of Obstetrics and Gynecology* 121 (1975): 707–13.
"What You Should Know about 'The Pill.' " *Journal of the American Medical Association* 213
    (1970): 1257–58.
Whitson, Leland G., Robert Israel, and Gerald S. Bernstein. "The Extrauterine Dalkon
    Shield." *Obstetrics and Gynecology* 44 (1974): 418–23.
Wilbur, Amy E. "The Contraceptive Crisis." *Science Digest* 94 (1986).
Wilensky, Robert J., and T. Brannon Hubbard, Jr. "Thrombosis of the Digital Vessels
    Secondary to Oral Contraceptives." *American Journal of Obstetrics and Gynecology* 113
    (1972): 1137–38.
Willson, J. Robert, and William J. Ledger. "Complications Associated with the Use of
    Intrauterine Contraceptive Devices in Women of Middle and Upper Socio-
    economic Class." *American Journal of Obstetrics and Gynecology* 100 (1968).
Wollen, Anne Lone, Per R. Flood, Roar Sandvei, and Johan A. Steier. "Morphological
    Changes in Tubal Mucosa Associated with the Use of Intrauterine Contraceptive
    Devices." *British Journal of Obstetrics and Gynecology* 91 (1984): 1123–28.
World Health Organization. *Intrauterine Devices: Physiological and Clinical Aspects.* Geneva:
    WHO, 1968.
————. Special Programme of Research Development and Research Training in Human
    Reproduction. "Multinational Comparative Clinical Trial of Long-Acting Inject-
    able Contraceptives: Norethesterone Evanthati Given In Two Dosage Regimens
    and Depo-Medroxyprogesterone Acetate. Final Report." *Contraception* 28 (1983):
    1–20.
————. Task Force on Intrauterine Devices. Special Programme of Research, Develop-
    ment and Research Training in Human Reproduction. "PID Associated with
    Fertility Regulating Agents." *Contraception* 30 (1984): 1–21.
Wright, Frank C. "Tuboovarian Abscess Associated with Laparoscopic Tubal Cau-
    terization and the Intrauterine Contraceptive Device." *American Journal of Obstetrics
    and Gynecology* 119 (1974): 1133–34.
Wright, J. T. "I.U.D. and Hydrorrhea." *British Medical Journal,* September 29, 1973, 696.

Wright, Nicholas H. "Infection and the I.U.D." *Obstetrics and Gynecology* 43 (1974): 923.

Yoonessi, Mahmood, Kent Crickard, Ivonne S. Cellino, Sateesh K. Sachidanad, and Wolfgang Fett. "Association of Actinomyces and Intrauterine Contraceptive Devices." *Journal of Reproductive Medicine* 30 (1985): 48–52.

Young, Warren R. "Beyond the Pill." *McCall's*, March 1967.

Zipper, Jaime A., Howard J. Tatum, Laura Pastene, Mario Medel, and Mirta Rivera. "Metallic Copper as an Intrauterine Contraceptive Adjunct to the 'T' Device." *American Journal of Obstetrics and Gynecology* 105 (1969): 1274–78.

Zuckerman, James E., and Phillip G. Stubblefield. "E. Coli Septicemia in Pregnancy Associated with the Shield Intrauterine Contraceptive Device." *American Journal of Obstetrics and Gynecology* 120 (1974): 951–53.

Zussman, L., S. Zussman, R. Sunley, and C. Bjornson. "Sexual Response after Hysterectomy-Oophorectomy: Recent Studies and Reconsideration of Psychogenesis." *American Journal of Obstetrics and Gynecology* 140 (1981): 725–29.

Index